Dedication

This book is dedicated to the Christie Ward, Vale of Leven Hospital, all of the Consultants, SHOs, nurses, staff, CPNs and GPs, along with all their staff, who have been and are involved with my care and to my friends and family who have always been there for me.

And finally to Lee and the others who fell by the wayside. You are missed.

It is out of respect and regard for those involved that their names have been changed.

Suzy Johnston
June 2004.

Acknowledgements and thanks

Sincere thanks to the **Scottish Association for Mental Health**, the **Renfrewshire Association for Mental Health**, ACUMEN (**Argyll and Clyde United in Mental Health**) and **The Bipolar Fellowship (Scotland)** for their financial help and unstinting support and to the **Scottish Executive's Mental Health Division's National Programme for Improving Mental Health and Well Being** and its 'seeme' Campaign for their encouragement and help regarding my ventures.

I am indebted to the following for all their help and assistance:

Mark Letham, Clydebank, (digital formatting)
Claire Letham, Clydebank, (artwork)
Simon Ashworth Photography, Helensburgh, (photograph)
Melissa Campbell, Helensburgh (The Cairn Logo design)
Everyone at the **Helensburgh Library** – especially **Fiona Sharkey.**

The Naked Bird Watcher

By

Suzy Johnston

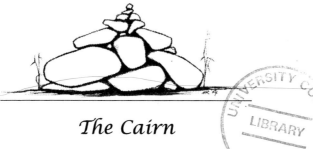

The Cairn

Copyright © 2002 Suzy Johnston

Updated 2nd edition published by The Cairn, August 2004.
The Cairn, Brincliffe, Dhuhill Drive West, Helensburgh G84 9AW,
 www.thecairn.com
First published by Chipmunkapublishing in 2003, copyright © 2002 Suzy
Johnston

A catalogue record of this book is available from the British Library
ISBN 0 9548092 0 3
Printed by Lightning Source UK, Milton Keynes, UK.

Suzy Johnston first became involved in mental health awareness programmes in 1999 when she joined the Education Team of the Renfrewshire Association for Mental Health. This followed her recovery from a series of episodes with severe depression that saw her hospitalised on numerous occasions. Giving talks to senior secondary pupils, social workers etc and writing about having mental illness for student psychiatric nurses, led to the publication of her autobiography 'The Naked Bird Watcher'. She is involved with The Scottish Executive's 'seeme' Campaign that addresses stigma and discrimination whilst raising awareness. Having written various articles and features, she researched and initially drafted the '1 in 4' Booklet for students on behalf of The Scottish Association for Mental Health and was encouraged to set up 'The Cairn' to publish, promote, write and advise on mental illness and its issues. For Suzy 'The Cairn' (the Scottish term for a pile of stones set as a landmark) symbolises the recovery from mental illness; the foundation stones being the support mechanisms helping to hold mental health in place – the support mechanisms being the network that is made up of either family, friends, colleagues or professionals.

She is also a musician/song writer and as an artist enjoys painting with acrylics.

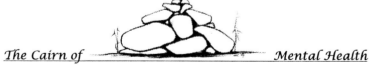

The Cairn of ————————————— Mental Health

The Cairn, Brincliffe, Dhuhill Drive West, Helensburgh G84 9AW Scotland
www.thecairn.com enquiries - info@thecairn.com

Foreword

It was in 2003 whilst he was Policy and Information Manager of The Scottish Association for Mental Health and editor of its magazine, 'The Point' that Simon Bradstreet wrote: "Accomplished athlete, recording artist, published author and manic depressive – Suzy Johnston isn't ashamed of any of her labels. In this candid and honest description of one person's experience of living a full and varied life at the same time as coping with a serious mental health problem, what continually shines through is the author's consistently positive outlook and her refusal to be ashamed of losing what she describes as 'the battle of percentages' in developing manic depression. In an engaging, informative and often amusing autobiography the author details the early onset of depression as a teenager but concentrates primarily on her university days, spent in St Andrews and lived in a typical 'work hard – play harder' student mode, interspersed with periods of disrupted study, relationship problems and psychiatric assessment. Whenever the story reaches a low point, following the ups and downs of the bipolar experience, there is often a funny anecdote around the corner. It is the author's ability to keep laughing in the face of diversity that marks this book out. One of Suzy's aims in writing this book was to help challenge the mindless and enduring stigma associated with mental health problems, pointing out that people who battle daily with mental health problems are worthy of applause rather than being discussed in embarrassed tones – as she puts it: 'bollocks to that!' With a determined spirit and forthright attitude Suzy Johnston is an example to everyone struggling to live with, or understand, serious mental health problems."

Simon Bradstreet is now Director of the Scottish Recovery Network.

CHAPTER 1

The sanity birds glided seamlessly through my dream, arcing high into the air on the updraft then swooping low over the churning sea. Again and again they completed their circuits, assured in their ability to navigate the wind's currents, revelling in their speed and dexterity, spreading reassurance through my body and calm through my veins.

Then one bird fell. Screaming, it dropped from the clouds, its body smashing into the hungry sea. Then another. And another, until the screaming was unbearable and even the clouds hurried to leave. The sky filled with death and the tortured cries of damned souls. The fear in the air was tangible and a dark, slick mass coated the sea that reeked of evil.

I sat bolt upright. The sweat on my body caused the sheets to stick to me. I looked at my right hand and then peeled the sticky sheet from my left hand and stared at it. They looked real but how could I be sure? All I knew now of reality was that I was a terribly evil person destined to burn in Hell. I was terrified, scared, petrified and I felt the bile rising in my throat.

"There is no way out of this." I mumbled to myself over and over; a sobbing mantra as I slowly rocked myself back and forward. I frantically racked my brain to find the evidence that condemned me to this fate but although the search was fruitless I still knew in my heart that I was a dreadful, dreadful person. I looked up at the clock that hung above the wooden door in the ward, it was 5:00am; too early to get up without attracting attention and the last thing I wanted was to speak to a nurse who, I had no doubt, would confirm my fears as she struggled to hide her disgust from me.

My eyes flicked over a picture of my family that was stuck haphazardly to my locker. I suddenly realised that if they found out how evil I was they would throw me out of the house and I believed that once they did I'd have to live in London and be penniless for the rest of my life. I would live destitute and alone, spending the days, weeks, months begging for scraps, lonely and frightened, rejected by those who had loved me. I felt the tears well up again in my eyes. "No!" I shook my head angrily as my inner voice shouted at me; tears were a dangerous a clue to others that something was wrong; I had to be in control or else everything would fall apart. I had to hide my evilness from the World until I found out a way of dealing with it.

These nurses and doctors were kidding themselves that I had manic depression. It was all lies. I was a fraud. An evil, repulsive fraud. I would be safe if I could somehow get myself discharged from this psychiatric ward. I knew that the nurses were talking about me behind my back and that some of them harboured thoughts of harming me. I had to get away. I had to get away.

CHAPTER 2

It bothers me somewhat that I have absolutely no recollection of the first three years of my life. Can you imagine what it would be like if you could remember every instant from being born and taking your first breath of de-toxified hygienised hospital air, to seeing your parents for the first time, to realising that bladder and bowel control were realistic targets with valuable social overtones and not just a way of gaining your parents' attention?

No one bothered to tell me at this time of conscious revelation (or if they did I was too busy discovering my toes to pay much attention) that life increased in complexity as one increased in years. I spent my early years in an immensely secure, nurturing environment unaware of my fortune in doing so and assuming that everyone else started out in similar fashion. Naivety can be a beautiful thing. I find it extremely ironic that we arrive in this world in perfect harmony with ourselves void of any demands other than survival and that we are perfectly happy in this state until our external environment informs us that this should not be the case. The world has much to offer – material wealth, power and social status and it seems to be human nature to run from what was originally perfect in order to chase our tails in an attempt to attain what society deems as perfection. There is no way of negating this trap, if indeed it is a trap. We are here to live our lives and it appears that to do otherwise would be a blatant rejection of natural law and society. Standing still is not permitted. As such we all do the best we can, leaving our innocence and naivety behind and replacing them with experience and knowledge.

Obviously, the environment in which you spend your formative years is of great relevance in indicating how you will turn out.

The sun threw out vivid colours as a form of goodbye as it went about the business of setting on a warm July evening in 1982. Cries of laughter and shouts of joy pervaded through the air as my two brothers and I played a game of football in the summer warmth with rules well beyond adult comprehension.

This is how I remember my childhood. Whenever I look back to those times I am comforted by a memory of happy days spent playing at home or at friends' houses and enthusiastically learning in school. I loved my life and I loved my family. Of course, it wasn't perfect, no one's life is. I had my fair share (some would say more than my fair share) of scrapes and accidents. One September evening I was racing the boy next door on my bike (he told me his new bike was faster than mine was). My elder brother Kit was the referee whilst my younger brother Ollie, who was four at the time, was appointed to the position of audience. I tore down the road pedalling as fast as I could, faster, faster, faster, my hair streamed backwards and my eyes watered in the wind. As far as I am aware the race was going well until the point that I lost control of my speeding bike and was flipped over the handlebars headfirst into an old but very robust brick wall.

I lost consciousness and landed in a forlorn heap, my stricken bicycle on top of me.

Kit was the first to react.

"Suzy!" he screamed, tears pouring down his cheeks. He ran towards me, battered trainers slipping in the muddy grass and grazing his knees as he dropped down beside me.

"Suzy!" he called again but more softly this time as he gently lifted my bruised head.

He turned to Ollie,

"Get Mum!" he shouted, "Ollie, get Mum!".

Ollie stood pale faced and unsure of what he was supposed to do. Slowly he turned and started jogging down the street towards our house.

"Run!" yelled Kit, his cry muted by the sobs that were shaking his small frame. Ollie started sprinting.

By the time he reached the house he was out of breath and arrived to find Mum in the kitchen and on the telephone

"Mum!" he gasped "Mum, Suzy needs you!".

My Mum motioned for him to be quiet; she was on the phone.

"Mum!" panted Ollie.

Covering the mouthpiece with her hand my Mum hissed " Ollie! Go and watch TV next door, I'll be with you in a minute!".

Obediently, Ollie traipsed through to the sitting room, sat down and started watching the TV. Cartoons were on. More specifically He-Man was on and Ollie was a great admirer of He-Man. Soon he was engrossed and didn't hear Mum enter the room.

"What was it about Suzy?" she asked.

No reaction from Ollie.

"Ollie. What did Suzy want?".

Slowly, Ollie turned from the blaring screen, his four-year-old brain filled with the wonder of dragons and fighting tigers.

"Uh…. Suzy's dead Mum. Suzy's dead."

I ended up with a concussion and a three-day stay in Hospital. Although I fully recovered I was left, in the short term, with some memory loss and somewhat

bizarrely, perfect aim. All this resulted in dramatic failure in the end of term book test– I couldn't remember the title never mind the story

- and an equally dramatic promotion to the position of goal shooter in the netball team, which lasted a few weeks until my usual scoring abilities returned.

My life trotted along quite merrily for a few years after this – I was good at my school work, made friends easily and had a family that I was close to. I had been informed at the age of nine that I had a talent for the game of squash, I began playing the sport seriously (well, as seriously as one does at the age of nine), becoming Scottish Under 14 champion with comparative ease. Basically I was happy. My family was happy. My life was moving along quite nicely and my future was looking very bright indeed. I was thirteen years old and about to receive a rude awakening that would have tremendous repercussions on the development of my personality.

I awoke one Monday morning, after returning from a squash tournament the evening previously, to discover that I was unable to move without exhaustive effort and excruciating pain; breathing was also a problem as were distorted vision, stuttering and shooting pains in my head. I was terrified.

After endless tests and a three day scare for my parents when the leukaemia test came back unclear (they didn't tell me about that until much later – my white cell count was through the ceiling) I was diagnosed as suffering from an unknown virus that was affecting both my brain and my body's general physiology. The doctors were non-committal as to my chances of recovery stating that "each case is different" whilst muttering "it's unusual to see this in someone so young". I spent seven months in bed before gradually returning to school and a further three years dealing with the longer-term effects before finally escaping the condition at the age of sixteen.

14

The experience is one that changed my life. Facing possible death or permanent paralysis at the age of thirteen has a way of making you grow up incredibly quickly. I was dragged out of my little, protective bubble realising I could never return whilst discovering that I didn't want to.

I was constantly being faced with people who would come to visit that were quite prepared to sit and sympathise for hours about how cruel life was and how terrible it was that I might never walk unaided again. "Isn't it a dreadful shame" and "I feel so sorry for you" were phrases I heard time and time again. My anger and refusal to lie back and accept my lot startled and I think in a way *offended* several people. Thankfully, my family understood my frustration and accepted my attitude, allowing me to push myself as hard as I could and they were there both for the successes and to offer support and consolation in the instances that I failed. I'll always be in debt to them for that.

Spending seven months in bed incapable of any physical exertion after being an extremely active person is a very trying experience. The initial frustration is immense and this is followed by a state of genuine exercise withdrawal in which the desire to get up and do something, *anything* is almost overpowering

I spent a lot of time lying in the dark, unable to sleep and listening to the noises that our old house makes as its wooded structure quietened down for the night. Those were long nights and I would spend considerable time thinking about all sorts of things; the future, relationships with the people in my life, attitudes, ideas, religion, hopes and dreams. As I lay there, month after month, external worries and fears faded as they became surplus to requirement. I became very analytical as I began to exercise my brain as I had once exercised my body and I had the time to sift through

my life experiences and squeeze every last drop of value out of them. By the time I returned to school my outlook on life, its philosophies and my expectations of it had changed greatly. I do not mean to imply that I was suddenly "worldly wise" and lived in an enlightened state - quite the contrary in fact. Questioning things that I previously had accepted as non-negotiable was both daunting and confusing. Life isn't simple, I guess if it was we'd have it all figured out by now, all I hoped for was that I had become more open minded and that I had escaped from the "padded cell", protective bubble in which I was previously immersed.

Depression first cast its despairing shadow during my final year at school; I was seventeen years old. I came into school that morning feeling, well, *strange.* It was as though the rest of the world had become muted and I felt void of any feeling. I found myself unable to communicate other than by a grunted yes or no – following conversations was impossible as I found the rich tapestry of words beyond my understanding. It was as if thick sheets of glass had been placed around me and I had no fight in me to escape, I was numb and the only emotion that I was left with was misery. I dragged my body around the school and presented myself at my classes but I might as well not have been there, I took nothing in and did not contribute. All the time I was swimming in a circle of darkness dully looking for some form of escape, I was confused, bewildered and desperately, desperately lost.

Then it passed. Just like that. Suddenly I was fine again and hurriedly forgot those bleak few days eager to convince myself that nothing was wrong, at the same time frightened to dwell on the recent past in case those dark feelings returned. I had no space in my life for depression. I was young and enthusiastic about life and my marks at school indicated the promise of a bright future. A mood disorder just didn't make sense. It made no sense at all.

I found sixth year a bit of a strain academically; I was studying subjects that I didn't particularly enjoy – chemistry, physics, maths and computing - but required in order to gain entry to St. Andrews University. In fact I doubt if I would have got the necessary grade in maths if it hadn't been for the help and support of my superb maths teacher, Mrs Hayes. Mrs Hayes spent hours of her free time patiently tutoring me and gently nudging me in the correct mathematical direction. We came to know each other fairly well during this period and upon leaving school she became a wise and trusted friend; someone I could turn to regardless of the situation.

In other ways my final year at school was a lot of fun; I was vice captain of the girls' hockey team and thoroughly enjoyed playing the position of goalkeeper. We took the opportunity to go on tour to Germany and had a fantastic time. The Youth Hostel that we stayed at endlessly served cheese and sausage regardless of the hour and dealt with our rather lame attempts to be funny in German with good humour. As for our free time, we went clubbing, hooked up with a Hungarian tramp who insisted on singing us the Hungarian national anthem and I was chased down a street by a panting shop owner for shop lifting (not guilty). We also managed to squeeze in three excellent games of hockey and unanimously declared the tour a great success.

We nearly managed to give our two hockey coaches the slip in the airport on the return journey as they were in Duty Free and hadn't heard the announcer call our flight early. Two of my friends, Wendy and Anna, and I raced into Duty Free to try to convince the two ladies that our flight really was boarding and that we weren't winding them up (as if we would). Eventually and on the third and final call they allowed us to drag them onto the plane where we were greeted by a polite smattering of applause by our other teammates.

School, generally, was pretty enjoyable although, of course, there were times in lessons when you would swear that the clock was running backwards and the class was never going to end. I'm sure there is some theory in physics that explains why time can run so achingly slowly when you're doing something that you don't enjoy and yet zoom by when you're having a good time. Beats me.

We were fortunate as a year in that we got on well with the staff. I don't mean that we sucked up to them, we just got on well and mutually respected each other. This made school a happy place to be; I remember that during our final Summer term one of the English teachers threw a party for us in a barn beside her farm house, both sixth year pupils and staff turned up and we had a great evening. It's funny, every time I hear the song "I Want That Man" by Debbie Harry I'm transported back to that night, jumping up and down with my friends in a big circle yelling the words, not caring whether they were right or wrong, spinning round and laughing, laughing, laughing.

School, for me, ended in June 1990. Now began the agonising limbo of no longer being at school but not knowing whether I had gained the grades required to go to University. So I decided to do the sensible thing: run away from it all. I booked a holiday in Majorca with some friends from school – Paul, his girlfriend Donna and Maggie- and my elder brother Kit. We spent five glorious weeks comparing tans and nursing sunburn, letting all the information that we had so conscientiously studied for our exams dissolve in the sunshine. Before we knew it it was time to return home to Scotland and meet with our respective futures face to face.

I was never any good at opening envelopes and this one from the Scottish Examination Board wasn't going to give up its contents without a fight. I continued my struggle, cursing under my breath, while my parents waited in the next room priming themselves to offer either congratulations or solace. Eventually I removed the slightly battered certificate from the battle-scarred envelope, I paused…. this was really it, the moment that would tell me how I would be spending the next few years. I decided to get this over with as quickly and humanely as possible, my eyes scanned the piece of paper. I had done it. I had done it! I was going to St. Andrews University. Bloody Hell.

CHAPTER 3

The town of St. Andrews was created in the 6th Century when it was known as Kilrymount; it gained its current moniker in the 12th Century when the remains of Saint Andrew were brought to the town to be buried at the Cathedral. All that remains of the Cathedral now is a collection of spectacular ruins that dominate the town's skyline when the sun fades into the horizon. St. Andrews itself is a beautiful, picturesque seaside town full of old buildings, winding lanes and cobbled streets. The lengthy stretches of sand that hold back the chilly North sea stretch out from the town like long protective fingers that beckon day trippers on hot Summer days.

I had visited St. Andrews in my sixth year at school to play in a hockey tournament there. All I had really seen of the town was hockey fields and changing rooms, so before we left for the journey home I ran down to the Scores and climbed up onto a railing in order to get as good a view of the beach as possible. It was glorious, and as I stood there with the wind whistling in my ears I made the decision that this was where I wanted to go to University.

My eyes squinted in the sunlight as I stepped out of the car on a clear September afternoon. The drive to St. Andrews had taken two hours and my nerves and excitement grew with each passing minute. I had tried to remember certain landmarks on the journey so that my future self could look at them and recall the emotion that I had been feeling at the time; kind of like an emotional Polaroid, something valuable to add to my collection of memories.

"Guess we better get the stuff out of the car." My Dad's voice broke my reverie. The car boot sprang open, eager to be rid of its load.

" Suzy, go and pick up your room key then come back and give your Mum and me a hand!"

I jogged down the street towards a large 19th Century terraced building that I had only minutes earlier discovered was McIntosh Hall, my home for the forthcoming academic year. I dodged in and out of the myriad of students and delivering parents that filled the road, the air filled with a haze of voices punctuated with shrieks of joy as returning students caught sight of old friends eager to catch up on what had happened over the Summer break.

I entered the Hall through a large wooden double door and joined a line of nervous and, as a result, very chatty First Years. I introduced myself and was met by a barrage of names that I embarrassingly immediately forgot and then enthusiastically exchanged will o' the wisp ideas of what courses we planned to take. Eventually I reached the head of the queue.

"Name please" uttered a small, thin man with a neatly trimmed beard and wire rimmed glasses.

"Uh…Suzanne Johnston"

"Let's see….room A24, here's your key. Can I have a £10 deposit please?"

"Sure, hang on a minute." I reached into my pocket and pulled out a tired looking £10 note. I handed it over to him.

"If you lose your key there are master keyholders, one on each floor, who will let you into your room. Come and speak to me if you still can't find it and I'll sort you out with a replacement, okay?"

"Okay, thanks." I picked up my key and headed back out to the car.

It took myself, Mum and Dad a good half an hour to carry my bags up to A24 which turned out to be on the top floor, but boy, was the view worth it. My room looked out over the world famous golf course and West Sands beach where I could see the waves tirelessly roll in and crash spectacularly on the wet sand.

I bade my parents farewell and hurriedly closed the door on my Mum's almost tearful goodbye; I looked round the large room with its wooden bureau, bed, sink, chest of drawers and single bed. Well, I was here. Guess I'd better unpack.

The first week of Winter Term at University is called Freshers' Week and what this means is that there are no classes as the student's spend their time registering for classes, meeting course tutors and consuming large quantities of alcohol with the security of knowing that there are no lectures to get up for the next day. Freshers' Week, legend has it, is when you make loads of new friends and spend the rest of the year trying to lose half of them! I'm not sure about the latter part of that sentence but the former is definitely correct; First Years in particular are eager to meet new people and make friends and the large amounts of beer swilling around make that process even easier.

I had come to St. Andrews with the security of knowing that five friends from school had also come to the University, but as they were all in different Halls from me I was surprised at how little I saw of them. This, however, was not a problem as I was fortunate to be in a Hall that had some great people staying in it, people that would become friends for life.

During Freshers' Week the Athletic Union runs trials for all of the University's sports teams and I was keen to be involved. Some of my new friends had also expressed an interest in joining the hockey club and trying out for the hockey team so five of us climbed on our bikes

23

and headed off for the Athletic Union. At this point I feel I should make the reader aware of another thing that occurs during Freshers' Week - everyone is trying to make friends, fit in and appear reasonably cool. I had been doing okay with this but unfortunately no one had told me how hard it is to ride a bike whilst holding hockey gear and just as we were cycling down the road to the A.U. I completely lost control and veered headfirst into a hedge. This embarrassing event was made worse by the fact that I was totally STUCK and required assistance to free myself. My friends were crying with laughter and any semblance of cool that I may have had dissipated into the air. Ah well!

After we had changed into our hockey gear in a busy and noisy changing room my friends and I jogged nervously round to the hockey pitch which, a helpful notice board informed us, was at the rear of the A.U.. Around sixty girls holding hockey sticks stood around in a rough semicircle at one end of the hockey field, at the centre of this crescent were ten students wearing St. Andrew's University tops – pale blue and white quarters. These girls were apparently in charge of the selection process and, amid a lot of laughing and joking, were taking down names on a clipboard.

A tall slim team member turned to me.

"Name?"

"Suzy Johnston"

"Position?"

"Goalkeeper"

"Ah, excellent; we're running a bit short on goalies. Go and get padded up, you'll find the equipment in that bag over there." She motioned to a muddy kit bag with a long willowy arm.

It turned out, in actual fact, that I was the only female hockey goalkeeper in the University so competition for a place in the team wasn't exactly fierce. Nevertheless, I was still going to be nervous and I was determined to give as good a show of myself in future games as possible.

The final night of Freshers' Week came around surprisingly quickly; the week seemed to have flown by. I decided to spend the evening with my friend Sophie in the Union bar. Sophie was in excellent spirits as her boyfriend Richard was coming over from Glasgow for the night and, after spending six whole days apart, she couldn't wait to be reunited with him.

"He's bringing his friend Sam with him."

" Uh huh." I replied, struggling manfully to open a bottle of extraordinarily cheap wine.

"Did I mention that Sam's single? And very good looking."

"Heh heh... would that be an attempt at subtlety, Sophie? Shit! Bloody cork!" I swore as the cork disintegrated in my hands.

" Here let me help you." She took the bottle from me. " No, it's just that I was thinking you should keep your options open. Anyway, Sam's a really decent guy, so just wait and see, okay?"

We strolled into the heaving throng that was the Union bar and I stuck close to Sophie as she scanned the crowd searching for Richard.

" There he is!" she shrieked "Come on! Richard! Richard!"

Richard turned out to be about six-foot, dark haired and enthusiastically downing a pint of lager in only the way that those who have just passed the legal age for alcohol consumption can.

"Sophie!" he yelled after he'd finished his drink " Come here you little fox!"

Sophie's giggle was abruptly halted as Richard planted a huge snog on her. I stood rather awkwardly as they continued their embrace, not too sure where to look.

"I guess you're Suzy" mumbled a tall, blonde man

" Sorry?" I yelled. The noise in the bar was deafening.

" Are you Suzy?" he shouted.

I grinned. "Yup, that's me!"

"Uh…I'm Sam. Fancy getting a drink?"

"Pardon?"

"A DRINK! FANCY GETTING ONE?"

I looked at him and noticed the smile that was playing across his lips and in his eyes.

"SURE, I'D LOVE TO!"

By the end of the night several things had happened; no 1: Richard had passed out, no2: Sophie had thrown up all over Sam's trousers, and no3: Sam and I had decided that we'd like to see each other again.

"Can I call you tomorrow?" he asked as we scraped the puke off his jeans. Romance, I thought, is not dead.

"Yeah, that'd be great" I smiled "I'll try not to be busy."

"Ha ha yeah right!" he laughed " I'll speak to you tomorrow or else I'll be forced to drive over from Glasgow and pin you against that wall."

He pointed at the wall over my left shoulder.

"Captain Romance aren't you?"

"You better believe it." he grinned as he scratched his nose. "You better believe it."

CHAPTER 4

I groaned as my alarm clock suddenly leaped into life and began blurting some terrible Beautiful South song. I was into my third week at Uni and I was already beginning to realise that choosing a 9:00am lecture had not been one of my greatest ideas. Grumbling, I rolled out of my bed and staggered off to the shower. Once I had got dressed I made my way down to breakfast exchanging "Hi"s as I passed various friends.

"God, this is killing me. I can't take these nine o'clocks anymore." I moaned as I sat down next to Kim.

" Hey, don't worry" she smiled and licked her spoon "Only two and three quarter terms to go."

The subjects I had chosen for that year were Cell Biology and Genetics, Biology of Organisms, Psychology and Sport and Exercise Science; an interesting little quartet that, on the whole, I found pretty enjoyable. However, it was Sport and Exercise Science that was causing me some problems, as not only was it at 9:00am it was also way over the other side of town which meant that every morning I had to climb on my rusty bike and cycle through the dark and, as often as not, pissing rain to make it to class. Not a huge amount of fun. Still, I liked the subject and that just about gave me enough motivation to drag myself out of my cosy bed every morning. This was followed by a bare-knuckle cycle ride to make it to Biology on time and then a more leisurely journey to Psychology at 12:00. On most afternoons I was kept busy with tutorials or lab classes except for Wednesday, which was reserved for the various sports that the University offered, and Friday which was mine to do pretty much as I pleased.

Sam had been coming through from Glasgow every weekend and I spoke to him at least once every day on the phone. Things were going great – we shared the same warped sense of humour, he was gentle and understanding and I was gradually falling in love with him. I couldn't wait to see him every weekend and the days in between seemed to stretch interminably. We would send each other ridiculously stupid letters that I would read over and over and eagerly await at mail time

One weekend, around the seventh week of term, my brother Kit came to stay, he had heard about the alcoholic lifestyle that students lead and had decided that it would be rude not to try it out first hand for himself. With this in mind Kit, Sam, Kim and I made our way to the Union. As ever, the place was heaving with people and successfully gaining a barperson's attention required strategy and cunning. I needed the loo so I excused myself and headed off to the toilet, leaving Kit, Kim and Sam to get the drinks in. I don't recall being gone that long but by the time I had returned Kit had downed five pints of Guinness in quick succession and, impressively, was still standing.

"You okay?" I yelled

"Absolutely fine" he slurred in reply "C'mon, let's go dance!"

We left the bar area and, pushing through hoards of drunken, sweaty students, made for the 'Megabop' – a school disco affair run by students in the main hall of the Union. I must have stopped now and then to speak to friends because it was at this point that I completely lost sight of Kit. I figured that he was a big boy and would be fine by himself for a bit so I spent a while dancing in the 'Bop' with Sam. As the

night drew to a close Sam and I split up and began searching for him. I decided to look in the dark, rather seedy, nether regions of the 'Bop' and found Kit sprawling semi conscious with his arm around a shadowy figure.

"Hey Kit!" I shouted "Time to go home!"

He grunted and slowly picked himself up into a standing position. Holding out his hand he helped his lady friend to her feet and as the tiring disco lights illuminated her face I couldn't believe my eyes. Of all the thousands of girls in the Uni that he could have hooked up with Kit had to choose a girl that, not only lived in my hall, but also lived in the room DIRECTLY OPPOSITE. Bloody Hell. Normally when Kit picked up a girl for a one-off date I would deliberately avoid them for the following few weeks and in doing so escape any awkward "When's Kit going to call me?" type questions. But this was one was going to be tricky. Bugger.

Kit, Sam and I walked with Meredith back to McIntosh Hall, the brilliance of the stars mocking the orangey glow of the town's lampposts. As we climbed the stairs to the top floor I was suddenly aware of how tired I was and I grabbed Sam's hand for support. After Kit said goodnight and farewell to Meredith he collapsed in one of my incredibly uncomfortable chairs and promptly fell asleep, snoring loudly.

The following morning Sam and I awoke early and in time for breakfast. I raised my head off the pillow and blearily looked over at Kit; he was still sound asleep, sprawled carelessly over my chair. I smiled, he had always been able to sleep anywhere as a child and it was obvious that he had retained this ability. Gently I woke Sam.

"Coming to breakfast?" I whispered.

"Yeah, sure. D'ya think I should get dressed first?" he queried jokingly

"Probably a good idea." I chuckled "I'm not sure if the World is ready for the sight of

you in your boxer shorts yet this morning."

The straggling mess of limbs that was my brother moved, uttered a moaning sound, and then lazily flicked open an eye.

"Did someone mention breakfast?"

Amid much yawning we found our clothes and got dressed, and as the three of us were heading out of the door I was suddenly aware that there were quite a few people in the corridor. Some of these people were friends but most were acquaintances that may have seen Sam with me before but had probably never set eyes on my brother. It was as I was mulling this thought over that Kit stretched in the doorway and exclaimed

"Shit! My fucking back! Suzy, what did you do to me last night?!"

You can imagine how THAT looked……..

Sam and I had been seeing each other for around ten weeks when he decided to drop the bombshell that he didn't want to go out with me anymore. I was surprised, hurt and distraught; I had thought that things were going really well between us and being dumped was the last thing I expected. He broke the news in a fairly sheepish manner outside the Central Bar on a damp Friday night and fighting back tears I asked for his reasons. He said he couldn't give me any. Great. I stormed off down the street heading somewhere, anywhere, the tears threatening to burst through at any second. Sam climbed into his car and drove after me.

"Suzy, get in the car!" he shouted through the wound down window.

"Leave me alone." I mumbled, tripping on a loose paving stone.

"This is stupid, look, you're getting wet – let me at least drive you home"

"Piss off." Bastard.

After much shouting on both sides I eventually got in the car and let him drive me back to McIntosh Hall. As I sat there, the squeak of the windscreen wipers breaking the awkward silence I noticed how long my fingers looked in the staccato lighting of the street lamps. I pressed my wet cheek against the cold glass of the window and stared aimlessly at the passing pedestrians hurrying through the rain. I wondered speculatively how their evenings were, whether they were having fun, meeting friends or just heading home, completely unaware that my life had just fallen apart.

Sam's car pulled up outside my Hall and I hurriedly grabbed at the door handle.

"You okay?" he asked.

I will not cry in front of him. I will not cry.

"Yeah, sure, I'm fine. Goodnight Sam."

I ran up the stairs to the main entrance and, without looking back, closed the heavy, wooden door behind me. I stood there in my wet clothes for a few minutes in a kind of shock trying to assimilate what had just happened.

"Hiya Suz, fancy a cup of tea? Oh my God, are you okay? What's the matter?"

As Kim spoke I let go of the huge weight of emotion that had been building up inside me and the tears began to pour from my eyes. She came over and gently put her arm round me.

"Come on; God you're soaking. Let's get you upstairs and into some dry clothes. I'll make you the best cup of tea ever, promise"

Kim guided me slowly along the hall comforting me with her presence and protecting me from intrusive stares from the few people milling around with looks that could cut

glass. I'm not sure how we made it to her room or where I got some dry clothes from but the next thing I recall is sitting in her room nursing a cup of hot tea and a horribly clichéd broken heart. Kim was superb; she let me cry, rant , yell and cry some more without so much as batting an eyelid. She refilled my mug with tea.

"What I don't get" she said as she passed over the sugar "Is WHY he broke up with you – it just doesn't make sense, you guys were great together."

"I know, I know, I know" I sighed "I don't get it either"

"You know that you have to talk to him and sort this out, if only for your own piece of mind."

"Yeah" A wan smile crept onto my face " I'm knackered, this breaking up stuff really takes it out of you."

" Oh my God - a touch of humour, there is hope for you after all"
Kim grinned "Go and get some sleep, we'll talk more in the morning okay?"

I stood up and stretched, yawning I hugged Kim and let myself out of her room.

I awoke early the next morning and sat in my bed for a while mulling over what had happened the night before. As I made myself a cup of tea I realised that Kim was right and that I really should try and talk to Sam and try and make some sense out of this mess. I leaned on the window sill and stared out at the glorious morning view, the steam from my tea slowly clouding the glass. "Why?" was the question that rang in my head. Maybe if I understood things a little better from his viewpoint I might accept this situation. Or maybe I just wanted something concrete to be angry at; something to blame, something to pin all this hurt I was feeling onto. I finished my tea, pulled on a sweatshirt on top of my pyjamas, opened my door and there sitting in last nights crumpled clothes and eating a Pot Noodle was Sam. He looked up at me.

"Great, you're awake. Finally. I've been sitting out here for ages" he set aside his Pot Noodle and pulled himself to his feet. "Can I come in?"

"Uh…what?" I mumbled, somewhat staggered by this turn of events. Sam pushed past me into my room and, grabbing my hand, pulled me in after him.

"Nice outfit," he chuckled motioning at my pyjama and sweatshirt ensemble" Going somewhere special?"

"Wha..wha..what the Hell's going on Sam? What are you doing sitting outside my room at 8:00 in the morning? You rather unceremoniously dump me last night and then turn up like this, I don't get you Sam, I just don't get you."

"Look, I just wanted to make sure that you were okay, I don't want us to part on bad terms – I like you too much for that."

"Sam, I'm confused. If you like me so much why did we have to break up?"

Wearily, Sam sat down on my bed. I could see a thousand thoughts cross his face and I knew instinctively that none of them was going to be the answer that I wanted to hear. He sighed, stood up and walked over to me.

"We just had to Suz, we just had to." And with that he took me in his arms and gave me a huge hug. A spark of hope jumped into life in my heart but I quickly damped it down. Sam, I realised, had his reasons and whatever they were he wasn't going to share them with me. I pushed him away.

"I think you had better go, I really can't handle this right now."

"Okay, I'm gone. Take care."

"Yeah, you too. Bye Sam."

He closed the door behind him and suddenly I was desperately alone in the room.

St. Andrews University is unique among Scottish Universities in that it runs an academic family system for its students; by this I mean that third and fourth years act as "parents" to first and second years. The purpose of this idea is to try and ensure that younger students, particularly Freshers, have an older, more battle-worn friend to turn to should any problems arise and it's also a skilful way of getting the years to mix with each other. A responsible parent will keep an eye on their "children", visit them regularly and help to make sure that they are enjoying the University experience.

But it's not all responsibility and helpfulness. Oh no. The main focus of the academic family comes at the end of the sixth week in first term in what is notoriously called Raisin Weekend. Raisin Weekend originally began as a civilised affair gaining its name from the bunch of grapes that were traditionally handed to the "father" as a gift which was followed by tea with "mother" and dinner with "father". However, this tradition, which I am sure was started with the best of intentions, swiftly mutated into an alcoholic feast of staggering proportions. As a first year I had heard all of the myths and urban legends surrounding Raisin Weekend – stories of students ending up unconscious and in hospital and rumours of people being arrested and kicked out of the University – so I approached the whole affair with a little trepidation but also, I confess, a lot of excitement. Raisin Weekend is really a misnomer – nothing much happens until Sunday afternoon and as I had been playing in a hockey tournament all day, alcohol had been strictly off the list. However, as we drove home in a rather seedy bus the older girls turned to us first years and recommended that we eat as much chocolate and drink as much milk as we could in order to line our stomachs. We sensed danger ahead. When we arrived home I quickly ran to my room, got changed into the pirate costume that my "father" had told me to wear and headed off to my "mum's" friend's house where the party was taking place. I arrived and quietly let myself in through the unlocked door all the while listening for the tell tale sounds of a party in full swing. There were none. Silence. I peeked into the living room and was met with a room full of very serious and sober people playing charades. This was not what I had expected.

"Uh, what's going on?" I whispered to my "mum", Kendra.

"I know, I'm sorry this party sucks, we were waiting for you to arrive before we left. Let me just grab Wendy and Dom and we'll be out of here. Oh yeah," she laughed "Nice Treasure Island outfit."

Kendra, Dom, Wendy and I ran through the driving rain and hurried into the welcome dry warmth of her kitchen. Once we had taken off our coats Kendra sat the three of us around her kitchen table and produced an unopened litre bottle of gin. She set it down on the table. "Okay, here's the game – each of you has a coin right? Right. You flip the coins in turn and the fourth person to land "heads" drinks two fingers of this lovely stuff, got it?"

"Straight gin? No tonic? Or lemon?" Wendy looked confused.

"Yeah! Don't worry, it tastes fine after the first few. Ladies and Gentlemen this is Raisin Weekend please commence the intake of alcohol. I've got some stuff to do next door – stuff for you guys for tomorrow – so I expect that bottle to be empty when I get back, okay?"

We began tossing the coins and started to fight our way through the gin. Sometimes people are lucky and sometimes they're not. This was not Wendy's night. She just kept losing – time and time again we would shout "Four heads" and it would be her hand reaching for the bottle. Dom and I got off fairly lightly but by the time the bottle was empty and Kendra had come back through Wendy was plastered. The door bell rang and a shout of "Where's my daughter?" cut through the gin induced euphoria that was beginning to envelope me. Kendra showed my "Dad" into the kitchen – he was wearing a ridiculous Captain Hook costume and the rain was beginning to smear his painted on beard.

"Wow, how much has she had to drink?" he nodded at Wendy who had fallen asleep at the table.

"Loads." I replied "C'mon, give me a hand to help her back to her place."

"No, no, it's okay, she can stay here. I'll look after her, don't worry about it. Get going to your "Dad's" party and have a good time – you

only have your First Year Raisin Weekend once. Now skoot!"
Kendra handed me my coat and started hustling me out of the door.

"Are you sure?" I called over my shoulder.

"Yup, absolutely. What do you think "Mother's" are for? If she's up to it we'll meet you in the Union later. Now go!" I gave Kendra a hug and followed my "Dad" out into the pouring rain.

Suffice to say my "Dad's" party involved more drinking – a particularly vicious punch if I remember correctly – and loads of inane party games which provided those partaking and those watching with a lot of laughs. At about 11:00pm the punch was finished, the games were over and it was time to follow the traditional path to the Union. I had had a great evening and was in high spirits as we showed our identity cards to the stewards in order to gain entry. As we turned the corner into the main Hall my good mood froze and a sickening feeling of horror and concern swept over me like a cloud casting a shadow on an otherwise sunny day. Dozens of people lay on the beer soaked carpet, some unconscious, some vomiting and some absolutely incoherent. These were the casualties of a night of excess, a night where the incentive to consume as much alcohol as possible often completely outweighs the body's capacity to cope. These people weren't alcoholics or irresponsible and in most circumstances had probably just hugely underestimated their capacity for booze, trying to impress their newly acquired families with their drinking abilities. A young man staggered towards me, mumbled something and, weaving past me, headed for the front door. I turned my head and followed his path with my eyes outwardly worried that he was okay, inwardly relieved that it wasn't me that had ended up in that state. He struggled to open the front door, made it out onto the street where, like a puppet whose strings had been cut, he collapsed on the pavement cracking his head on the ground.

"Oh my God!" I cried, a sickening lurch in my stomach mixing uneasily with all that I had consumed that evening. "Quick! Help him! Help him!"

I stood rooted to the spot, outstretched arm pointing, faintly aware of the stewards rushing past me and out the door.

"Suzy c'mon, there's nothing you can do." My "Dad" hugged me, my shaking arm still pointing towards the horrific scene. "Look, they've called an ambulance. Let's go inside." I allowed myself to be bustled inside, stepping over the nameless bodies lying on the floor. I allowed myself to meet up with my friends. I allowed myself to have a

good time. And I allowed myself to forget about that young man because it was easier to forget than to admit to myself that if I had helped him instead of silently judging his state of debauchery he might not have fallen. The party was over, it was time to go home.

In accordance with the ancient and somewhat bizarre traditions of the University the following morning was spent being dressed up in ridiculous costumes by our mothers and then taking part in an Enid Blyton style shaving foam fight in St. Salvator's Quad – silly, juvenile and extremely good fun. As I walked back to my Hall through the streets of St. Andrews I was filled with a sense of belonging; as though I was now truly a part of the University. Raisin Weekend had served its ultimate purpose. I smiled to myself as I climbed into the shower, the traumas of the previous night forgotten; I had never been happier.

January has always been a cold, dark way to start the New Year and the beginning of 1991 was no exception to this rule. The trees shivered as the rasping wind toyed with their fragile branches and the grey, overcast sky hinted at the promise of snow later in the day. I shuddered as I pulled my heavy coat close around me and buried my chilled face deep into the familiar warmth of my old school scarf. It was the 6th January and I had just turned 18 two days ago; it was the first day of the new term and I was determined to spend the evening celebrating my birthday with my friends. I hurriedly made my way down the street to McIntosh Hall, the artificial lights at the window shouting sanctuary from the freezing elements and climbed the old, worn steps up to the front door.

"Hey Polly! Are you back yet?" I yelled as I walked along C-floor unbuttoning my jacket. Polly's door flew open and a medium build dark haired girl stepped into the corridor.

"You betcha! How are you? How was your holiday? Miss me much?"

"Uh….I'm fine and absolutely ready to consume an obscene quantity of alcohol. Miss you? Who are you again….?"

Polly chuckled and took my arm.

"C'mon in, I'm still unpacking as you can see" Polly's room was a jumble of clothes, bags and hockey equipment "So when do the celebrations begin? I feel that as an extremely responsible 22 year old I should be involved from the start."

"Well, Michelle, Winnie, Lesley, Carl, Kim, John and Ann are coming round to my room at 7:00pm for champagne." Polly looked at me.

"Okay, fizzy wine. Then we're heading out to the pub to meet up with Emily, Angie and the others. Who knows where the evening will lead from there?"

Much, much later I careered to a staggering halt outside my room and fumbled in my pocket for my keys. In the immense wisdom of youth my friends and I had decided that as it was my 18th birthday I had to consume eighteen drinks, so that six glasses of wine and twelve vodkas later I was feeling very much the worse for wear.

"Kim can you find my keys; my hands aren't working" I slurred.

"I'm not sure if mine are either. I'll try." she said reaching into my coat. "Here we go."

She opened the door and we stumbled inside.

"Hey! It's my bed! I love my bed!" I collapsed onto my duvet and felt waves of

drunken tiredness overwhelm me. I closed my eyes.

"Polly, are you still there?"

"Yeah, I'm here – I'm just getting you a glass of water. Heh, heh I think you might need it."

"I love you guys. I just need to sleep and I'll be fine."

"Okay g'night Suz. See you in the morning."

"Okay, night Kim, night Polly see you bright and perky in the morning. Bright and perky, bright and perky la la la " I hummed to myself.

Surprisingly, I made it to breakfast the next day but, boy, did I feel like death. I sat on my own and, trying to ignore the swirling nausea in my stomach, optimistically nursing a glass of milk. Julie, a third year I was getting to know, plonked herself down beside me.

"God, you look terrible. Are you okay?" she enquired.

I managed a weak smile.

"Actually, I think there's a strong possibility that I might not make it to lunchtime."

"Heavy night last night?"

"Extremely." I wiped a light sweat from my brow.

Actually, I kind of wished that Julie would go away and leave me alone; I was finding it hard to concentrate on our little conversation and still manage to keep the bile from continuously rising in my throat.

"Have you been sick?"

"Uh, yeah. About nine times."

I had spent half the night on my knees and the other half wending my way between the toilet and my room, occasionally pausing to rest my face against the welcome cool of the corridor wall.

Julie put an arm round me and squeezed.

"Look, my room's between yours and the loo, next time you have a night like that knock on my door on the way past."

I lent into Julie's hug.

"Thanks Julie, that's really sweet."

"Yeah," she grinned wickedly "I'll bring my camera, it'll be great!"

You would have thought that four continuous days of vomiting would have taught me a hard lesson about the perils of alcohol but no, I proved to be a student of the particularly stubborn variety and blithely put my unpleasant stint of alcohol poisoning down to that infamous "bad pint" that so many drinkers speak of. Drinking was and is a huge part of University life; many friendships are bonded over a pint of lager or six and alcoholic excursions are at the centre of most University clubs' social calendars. I would guess that I spent about five evenings a week with friends in one pub or another in my second term at St. Andrews and, whilst my work definitely suffered as a result, I do not regret that time in the slightest as the friendships I

41

made and the memories I forged are worth more than any exam score that I might have otherwise achieved.

All in all I was enjoying the student life – I had made some great friends and I was finding the subjects that I was studying absorbing and interesting. During my first term I had studied hard as I was unsure what was expected of me and, as a result, aced my exams. I decided to let things slide a little bit in second term, just enough so that I would still obtain my exemptions – exemptions from the big degree exams in third term – but also enough so that I could relax a little and have a bit more fun. Life was for living.

CHAPTER 5

If life had been simple I would have woken up one day, said "Oh my God. I'm depressed." and gone to the Doctor and been given some pills that would make me better. Clean cut, decisive, and uncomplicated. Perfect. But life is never that simple, and I didn't have a clue what was happening to me. This wasn't a depression that landed on me, full force, out of the blue. Oh no. This depression was sneaky and insidious, gradually working its way into all facets of my life, gradually removing every bastion of self-worth and self-confidence that I had. I started losing my capability to concentrate; I would read a chapter of a book and all the pieces of information would fall out of my head like leaves in an Autumn storm, frantically I would read it again but to no avail. Fucking hell, what was happening to me? As the University began its third term I began finding it increasingly difficult to leave my room, to hold conversations with people, to remember to eat and to wash myself. Previous feelings of joy and excitement were being replaced with dread and fear and I would spend hour upon hour, day and night, lying on my bed staring at the ceiling looking for I don't know what. I was so confused by how I was feeling and the idea of explaining it to anyone seemed preposterous; after all, if I didn't understand what was going on how could anyone else? I was completely absorbed by this dark, murky, all consuming world and I failed to notice that the real world was rushing by – it was Summer, people were falling in and out of love, there were parties on the beach, and the smell of fresh cut grass in the air.

I took part as best I could. I really did. It's just that there seemed to be a kind of thick opaque film over everything that made it impossible for me to see or feel things

properly. I felt nothing when a bunch of us sat on the beach and watched the sunset, I felt nothing when I tried to comfort an upset friend, and I felt nothing when my boyfriend kissed me. I was becoming more and more removed from reality and I was getting increasingly scared because it all felt so out of control.

I decided one afternoon to try and talk to Max, my boyfriend of two months, about how I was feeling, desperately hoping that he would somehow sort out the mess in my head and make the world right again. I knocked on his door.

"C'mon in, it's open!" I walked into his room and closed the door behind me.

"Heya Max, how're you doing?"

"Good thanks. You?" he looked up from the book that he was making notes on. I picked up a CD that was lying on his duvet and pretended to read the tracklisting.

"Oh you know, okay I suppose" Liar.

He pushed his notes aside "D'ya fancy getting out of here and going for a coffee?"

I was shocked at how nervous I felt about disclosing to Max how I was really feeling, I mean he was my boyfriend, my partner for goodness sake. Maybe I should leave. Maybe I should try and sort this one out on my own. I've never liked showing weakness to people and that's what this amounted to. Oh God! What to do! I read the tracklisting on the CD again, backwards this time.

"Uh, no. Let's stay here, there's something I want to talk to you about."

"Oh, okay. What's up?"

I felt so vulnerable and in my mind's eye I saw myself shrink to about a centimetre tall.

"It's just that, well, it's just that I haven't been feeling so good recently." I stumbled over my words. Max frowned.

"How so?" he asked

How do you tell someone that you feel as though nothing matters anymore, that you're stuck in a hopeless void and that even breathing takes more effort than it used to? "How can you not see what is going on?" I wanted to scream, HOW CAN YOU NOT SEE? To me it was all to horribly obvious that something, somehow was wrong. This, I guess, was my big moment to eloquently and articulately explain what was going on in my head but apathy had been sucking on my veins for too long and I couldn't bring myself to really care.

"I've not been feeling too great recently; I'm not sure whether I'm stressed, depressed or ha ha just going mad and I don't know what to do." I closed my eyes and sat down on the bed.

"For real? No mucking around?" Max looked worried.

"For real. No mucking around." I suddenly felt really tired and I wished this conversation was over. Max stood up and began pacing round the small badly lit room. I lay down and took refuge amongst the pillows.

"How long has this been going on?"

"Sorry?"

"How long have you been feeling like this?" he asked

"I don't really know….about a month or so I suppose"

45

"So you've known for about a month and you decide to drop this on me now just as I have exams around the corner?"

"What?" I was startled "I'm sorry, I didn't think…I'm sorry"

"And anyway, what am I supposed to do about it? Do I look like a shrink? I don't

need a loopy girlfriend hanging around me right now." God, he looked mean.

"I just thought…"

"No, you didn't think. You're just too damn self absorbed – everyone has bad times but you get through it. You just need to pull yourself together." He suddenly dropped down on the bed beside me.

"C'mon babe, you know I care about you but this is really bad timing. Look, if it makes you feel better book an appointment to see your GP; she'll put your mind at rest. Okay? Okay?"

"Okay." I said in a very small voice. "I'd better be going now."

"Sure. Don't look so worried, you'll be fine. I'll see you at dinner."

As I pulled the door shut behind me the numbness that I felt in my head threatened to overwhelm the rest of my body. My "talk" with Max hadn't gone anything like I had expected it to – was he right? Was I being self-absorbed? Could I just pull myself together? Did other people feel this way? If so why had nobody mentioned it to me before? If they had maybe I might have been able to organise some sort of fight plan in advance and been able to beat this thing before it had got started. Or maybe not. I don't know. I felt so isolated, so powerless and speaking to Max hadn't helped at all, I just felt worse. God, I was so confused. I ran back to my room, pulled the curtains shut and locked the world out. Maybe I had to sort this out myself. Call the doctor? Surely that couldn't go any worse than the conversation I had just had with Max. There was something wrong, I told myself firmly, maybe a Doctor might be able to ease the pain I was feeling. Just as long as she didn't laugh at me or call me a waste of time. I didn't think I could handle that.

The doctor, Dr Boon, didn't laugh at me. She decided that I was suffering from stress even though I assured her that my forthcoming exam was meaningless to me and prescribed some beta blockers which had the effect of slowing down even further my already lethargic world. For the next week I lived my life in slow-mo stumbling from pillar to post in a haze of medication, the mental torment that I was suffering untouched by this wave of molasses that engulfed me. My Mum phoned to say that she and Mrs Hayes, my former maths teacher, were planning to visit the next weekend and would that be okay? "Sure!" I replied keeping my voice light but inwardly panicking at the thought of the impending meeting. I had told Mum about how I had been feeling over the past month or so but, as ever, I had been continually frustrated at my inability to express what was really going on. I was concerned because I was unsure whether I could keep it together for the whole weekend and besides, she was bound to pick up on the effect that the beta blockers were having on me. No, I thought I would tell her exactly what was going on in a calm, controlled manner and try not to alarm her. There was no point in both of us feeling bad. I had another appointment with Dr Boon booked for the following Monday so I could reassure her that my "situation" was being monitored.

As I walked towards McGregors' café the following Saturday morning, the grey weather matched my mood and I was unsure of what I was going to say. I felt particularly weak that day, whether because of the drugs or lack of sleep I wasn't sure, and I struggled to open the front door. I entered the café, my face wet from the rain, shrugged off my coat and looked around for my Mum and Mrs. Hayes. They

beckoned to me from an exposed table in the middle of the room and I gave them both a hug and sat down. I ran my fingers through my long, damp hair and absentmindedly tied it into a ponytail.

"Hi, how are you both?" I felt edgy and started to wring my fingers under the table.

" Good thanks. It's great to see you, God, you're soaked - is it still raining out there?" Mum asked.

"Yeah, it's pretty wet, uh, I'll have a white coffee please." A white shirted waitress hovered beside our table patiently awaiting our order.

"Cappuccino for me." said Mum

"And a black coffee for me please." added Mrs Hayes

"Thanks for coming over to see me Mrs Hayes, I'm glad you came. I miss our maths lessons, can you believe that?"

"I'm sure you do" she chuckled " And drop the Mrs Hayes bit, it's Isobel okay?"

I blushed "Okay….Isobel, so where are you guys staying?"

"At a B+B around the corner, I thought we might stop in Crail on our way home and I could show Isobel where I spent my Summer holidays when I was a kid. Fingers crossed the weather will be better than today." Mum said hopefully.

There was a lull in the conversation as the waitress served our coffees and I imagined for a moment that I was an ant, tiny and fragile with no power over my existence.

"Suzy?" Mum broke my reverie "How are things going with Dr Boon?"

"To be honest Mum, I'm not too sure, I mean she's started me on some pills but I don't think they're working."

"What sort of pills are they?" asked Isobel

"Beta blockers – I think they're to calm me down."

"And do they? Calm you down I mean?" Mum looked concerned, she hadn't touched her coffee.

"Yeah. Well they slow me down but I've been trying to explain that I don't think I'm stressed and I don't think I need to be calmed down."

"How are you feeling then?"

"Oh God, I don't know."

How to explain my dark, murky world to them? Talking about it was an admission that it was really happening and that made it harder to hide from. Running away from yourself is an exhausting process.

"You have no idea how much I want to tell you how I feel. I've spent hours going over this conversation in my head racking my brains desperately trying to find the right words. Don't you see? I'm an idiot. Useless. I feel so bad but I can't say why" I sighed. "I have this huge bleak emptiness that makes me ache inside. I've stopped being able to feel. I do things on automatic and making decisions becomes nearly impossible. Do you know that I sat for ten minutes this morning staring at my socks because I was unable to decide which one to put on first? You see this cup of coffee? I don't even know if I want it, I couldn't tell you I just don't know. I feel lost and I'm worried that I can't be helped."

"You know that I love you very much don't you?" Mum reached under the table and grabbed my hand.

"I know you do Mum, I know you do and I love you too. I'm sorry about all this."

"When are you seeing Dr Boon again?"

"Monday. I'll try to talk to her about this again. I don't think these pills are helping I

just feel spaced out on them and as I'm having my own problems connecting with reality I think I could do without that."

"Do you want me to stay on till Monday and see her with you?" queried Mum

"No, I'm fine seeing her on my own. Thanks though. I'll give you a call and let you know what's going on." There was a lull in the conversation and we all stirred our coffees contemplatively.

"How're Kit and Ollie?" I asked changing the subject.

"Fine, fine. Kit's doing okay at college and Ollie wants to come over to see you. What do you think?"

"It would be great to see him - I miss them both but let me sort things out with Dr Boon before we make any decisions about him visiting - I'd like to get my head sorted out a bit before I see him as I'm not much fun to be around at the moment and I'd like to be in a better mood when he's here."

"Maybe you could call him tonight?"

"Maybe. Maybe I will."

What was I saying? That wouldn't happen, at least not today anyway, I was too knackered from this conversation already. Time to leave. I drained my coffee and spent a few seconds distracted and absorbed by the pattern my coffee residue made in my cup.

"Suzy? You okay?"

"Uh yeah fine. Listen, if you and Isobel don't mind I'd quite like to go back to my room and catch up on some sleep. I'm just really tired. And I've kind of run out of conversation. Mum don't look so worried, I'll be okay."

"Hmmm. Okay look, you go and have a snooze and we'll come round and pick you up

for lunch at, say, 1:00. C'mon give me a hug and we'll talk more later."

As I left it was as though half of me sat and watched from the far corner of the coffee shop as the three of us stood up and exchanged hugs and only I caught the fleeting look of unhappiness that crossed my face as I opened the door of the cafe and headed out into the rain.

Anti-depressants. After our Monday morning appointment Dr Boon had put me on anti-depressants. Shit. What did this mean? Was I depressed? Was that why I couldn't eat, couldn't sleep, couldn't talk to people? I thought depressed people were supposed to feel sad and cry all the time. Not me. I didn't feel ANYTHING, I was an emotional mute and I didn't, couldn't cry. God knows I'd tried. In the dark secretive hours of the night I'd lie awake thinking of things to make me cry and been continually frustrated at my inability to squeeze out even one solitary tear. Crying would have been a relief, an escape from this deadness that I was feeling. I opened the pill bottle and tipped its contents out onto my hand. Thirty small red pills. Impressively unimpressive. If I closed my hand I could pretend that they weren't there and that everything was normal. I carefully poured them back into the bottle, leaving one in my hand. I stared at it for quite a while and when I poked it with my left forefinger I noticed that some of the red colour had come off on my palm. Quickly and before I changed my mind I popped the pill into my mouth and gently rolled it round with my tongue. It tasted sweet. Sugar coated reality. Hmmm. Was this what I wanted? What I needed? I stared hard into the mirror above my sink trying to see something that I hadn't seen before. Blonde hair, blue eyes, blank expression. Nothing new. I filled a glass with water and drank its contents, washing the small red pill into my stomach. Once again I stared

hard at the figure in the mirror "This is your fault." I thought "This is your fault. You should be able to beat this on your own. Why are you such a loser?" I turned from the mirror. It was 10:05am and I was late for my lecture.

The Summer holidays after my first year were difficult both for me and my family. I was struggling to get a grip on an illness that I didn't understand and my parents were baffled by my behaviour. I would spend hours lying on my bed staring at the ceiling completely preoccupied by the negative thoughts that trudged slowly round my brain. I was confused. Tired . Scared. I couldn't even begin to find the right words to explain this disastrous mess to my folks. I just wanted to be left alone in the absorbing, timeless void that was my head and try and think my way out of a hopeless situation.

I would have better days when I could talk with people, even laugh and joke but then the fog would close in and shut off any real attempts at conversation. I would become distracted and withdrawn. The World presented itself to me with a sense of unreality and I felt as though a thick glass wall surrounded me, forcing upon me a feeling of detachment and isolation. If I screamed no one would hear. My parents gently tried to encourage me to take part in everyday activities. "Come down town and do the shopping." "Phone one of

52

your friends.". Unfortunately they didn't understand at that time that when I was feeling depressed those things were impossible for me. I resented their quiet enthusiasm about life and felt even more alienated by it. Nobody else felt like this and I was beginning to believe that nobody could make me feel better. I would curse myself relentlessly, over and over, for thinking such dreadful thoughts and at times, when I had the energy, force myself to pretend that everything was okay-dokey-thanks-very-much. The things we do to run
away from ourselves.

To make matters worse I had a resit to do during the Summer holidays after spectacularly failing a Degree exam during the previous term and that was preying on my mind. I had never failed anything major before and if I didn't pass it this time around I would have to "carry" the subject next year. That thought wasn't too appealing. I was in trouble and it was obvious even to me that I wasn't coping.

I had started seeing a psychiatrist, Dr Paisley, at the end of the previous term, a concept that I was both alarmed and encouraged by. Alarmed in that "did this mean I was mad?" and encouraged that things might start to improve. When I entered his office at the end of an unusually warm May I carried my depression with me like an ill-fitting overcoat that I was desperate to be rid of. I sat like a standard issue NHS patient on a standard issue NHS patient's chair and, as requested, began to tell him about my life. I felt worse as I did this as it became perfectly apparent to me, and possibly him, that I had had a great life and therefore had no excuses to hide behind for feeling the way I did now. I took a big deep breath and asked why was this happening to me – I am of the quick fix-it mould; find out what's causing the problem then sort it and everything will be okay. Unfortunately Dr Paisley had no direct answers to give and instead muttered darkly and confusingly about chemicals in the brain and faulty synapses. What?

After we had talked for sometime he reviewed my medication and decided to change me onto another anti-depressant that he hoped would work more effectively. I hoped so too.

My mood lifted as the Summer progressed and I did my best to convince myself that what had happened over the past few months was a one off, a "blip", a bad run that had knocked me off track but that would never happen again. Sure, I was still taking the medication but I knew that I didn't really need it and the sooner I stopped taking it the better. Everything was back to normal. I sat and passed my resit and I was greatly looking forward to the new academic year where I would be sharing a flat with three friends: two fourth year girls, Yvonne and Ruth and a third year bloke, Niles.

I moved into the house at the beginning of October 1991, gave Yvonne and Ruth a huge hug and, trying my best to ignore the swirly psychedelic carpet in the hall, started to unpack. Niles arrived later that day and we all sat round the wobbly dining room table for our first meal together (it was spaghetti bolognaise – true student fare).

The next morning the doorbell rang and the four of us went to answer it. On the doorstep stood a postman holding a very large box that had "Durex" stamped all over it in huge, red letters. The reason for this delivery was this: Ruth was running the AIDS Awareness stall at the Freshers' Fayre and she had talked Durex into donating loads of condoms to give away as freebies. This fact was not known by our new neighbours who were all out in their gardens staring, not too subtly in our direction. Niles took the box from the postie and then raised his voice and said " Aaaaah, this should do us for a couple of weeks at least. C'mon girls let's get back to bed."

As you can imagine, our reputation in the area soared.

Later that evening I was sitting in the pub with a group of friends, absentmindedly listening to Madonna telling us how to "Vogue" and quietly sipping a coke. It was the first night of Freshers' week and we were all delighted to be back in each other's company. Linda, a fourth year friend of mine, stubbed out her cigarette, drained her pint and lent towards me and said in a concerned manner "How come you're not drinking, Suzy?"

I looked down at the floor.

"I'm taking some medication just now and it's best that I don't drink"

"Hmmm, I see.....what sort of medication?"

I glanced up and realised that everyone at the table was waiting for my answer.

"Anti-depressants" I said quietly

"But you don't need..."

"What the Hell are you taking those for?"

"Hold it everyone " interrupted Linda " This isn't the best place for this conversation. Let's talk about it later. Anyone need another drink? It's my round."

If a large hole had opened up in front of me I would have gladly jumped into it head first. I felt mortified. I had laid open my failings for public inspection and I couldn't handle it. Why was it such a big deal? If I had said I was taking antibiotics for a nasty chest infection would I have gained such a reaction? I didn't think so. Why was it so hard for them to believe that one of their friends, one of their group,

55

might have had a mental health problem? Did they feel guilty because they hadn't picked it up earlier or was it that they wanted to dismiss it out of hand because only "other people" became mentally ill? I returned to sipping my coke as anonymously as possible and tried to put all of these questions out of my mind.

As Linda and Julie walked me home that night I was waiting for the onslaught but neither of them mentioned anything other than small talk until we got back to the house. It was when they came up to my room with me and sat on the bed that the grilling began.

"Why are you taking antidepressants? You seem fine to me." began Julie.

"I had a bit of a rough time last term and through the Summer break. I was feeling really low, but yes, I do feel better now." I replied

"Hey, everyone gets a bit low sometimes but you don't need pills for that you just need to pull yourself together and get a grip."

"No, you don't get it! I had tried pulling myself together and nothing was happening.

I felt as though I was running out of options."

"So why didn't you come and speak to me?" asked Linda

"As stupid as it sounds it was because you were a third year and I was only a first year. I felt intimidated. Besides I was scared of talking about it. Talking about it made it seem more real."

"But you said you're feeling better now?" said Julie.

"Yes."

"Good, so stop taking the drugs, you don't need them!"

"My psychiatrist says I'm to keep taking them."

"Your what?"

"My psychiatrist." Please could everyone go away and leave me alone.

"Look Suzy" said Linda as she put her arm round me. "This has all got way out of hand, all you need is some good nights out with your friends – we'll keep you right. What are you going to do about the pills?"

"I'm going to keep on taking them. I really trust my doctor and, yes, the psychiatrist and if they say take them then I'll take them. Y'see you don't know how I felt and if taking a few pills means that I won't feel like that again then I'll go ahead and take them. Can we drop this now? Please?"

"Okay, but promise me you'll at least talk to us if you start feeling bad again, we're here for you, you know?" added Linda as she gave me a hug goodbye.

"I know, and likewise." I hugged her back

" I'm still not happy about these pills…" murmured Julie as she hugged me.

"I realise that but please understand that this is something that I need to do."

"Come round for lunch tomorrow, Suzy and we'll talk some more." said Linda as she pulled open my badly hung bedroom door.

"Good night both of you" I called after them as they disappeared down the staircase.

The first seven weeks of term-time flew by and I was having a great time; I was making new friends and enjoying and coping with my course work. Yes, I was still taking medication but I had almost managed to persuade myself that I would never be depressed again. I'd talked to Dr Paisley about the negative thoughts that I was sometimes still bothered by and he had again adjusted my pills but all in all things were good and I was once again unprepared for what life was about to throw at me.

CHAPTER 6

It was around the eighth week of term when the darkness started spilling into my life again and this time there was a new twist – hallucinations. One evening I was sitting in our living room studying. I looked up at the clock on the wall to check the time and somehow in that split second, when I turned my gaze back to my notes, I had lost the ability to read; the words and letters in front of me just appeared like a collection of squiggles. I shook my head and stared at the TV. At that point I was unaware that the TV was switched off because there appeared to be a black and white western on the screen. I looked closer. There was a bar room brawl happening but, completely out of place, there was a girl sitting on a sofa in the background. I gradually came to realise that the girl was me and as this realisation hit, large blobs started firing out of the TV towards me. I scrambled out of the room, ran upstairs and hid under my ever-protective duvet. What the fuck was going on? Was I losing my mind? I decided right there and then that I would not tell anyone about this. This would be my secret. I wasn't mad. I wasn't mad. Was I?

I was beginning to flounder in a world of negativity and trying desperately to hold things together and maintain an appearance of normality but the cracks were beginning to show. I was finding it increasingly hard to be social and putting on a front was becoming a life skill. Studying was becoming impossible as my brain steadfastly refused to absorb any of the facts presented to it and I was starting to panic as exams were just around the corner. Then one day I lost it. Completely.

I was in Yvonne's room talking about everyday things when suddenly I lost my grip and the façade of a happy "normal" student slipped from my grasp. I burst into floods of tears. I simply couldn't hold it together any longer and months of repressed emotion overwhelmed me. I tried to explain that I didn't understand what was going on in my head, that nothing made sense, that I felt lost. Yvonne tried to reassure me that everything would be fine and I tried to believe her, but I knew that this ran a whole lot deeper than just "a bad day" and I was becoming increasingly frightened. I didn't mention the hallucinations; I was scared of admitting them to myself, never mind someone else. I pulled together the shreds of survival personality that I had left, stopped crying and awkwardly thanked Yvonne for her support. I realised that something was going to have to change and that studying at University was not the right thing for me to be doing at that time. I would discuss it with my parents and my doctors but I had decided that I would have to "drop out" for a year. I was in no shape to study and if I was to claw back my health I needed some time to do it.

The following months were a horrible blur. Dr Paisley increased my medication as my state of mind deteriorated and I was left dealing with side effects that left me stoned and exhausted. My favourite time of day became night time when I was in a medication induced sleep as at least then I could escape from the terrible thoughts and feelings that tormented me. There was so much going on in my head and I was able to articulate only a tiny portion of it. I became frightened of my flatmates and I was sure they hated me so I shut myself away in my room and tried to stay out of their way. I was becoming increasingly confused and the hallucinations were becoming a regular feature. Still I struggled with presenting a façade of normality and continued to drag myself out of the safety of my house and meet friends for coffee. My friends were superb and encouraged me to talk about how I was feeling; they may not have had the answers that I was looking for but it was reassuring to know that they were there for me.

At other times communication became impossible and I began to wildly misinterpret what people meant when they spoke to me. One evening I was about to go bowling with some friends and I met Julie on the stairs as I came clattering down.

"What the Hell are you wearing?" she asked

I was wearing all black apart from a Hawaiian blue short sleeve shirt that I had on under a charcoal cardigan.

"Nothing...just let me go." I muttered

"No way! The others have got to see this! Come into the sitting room." She grabbed my arm and pulled me down the stairs. We entered the front room where Yvonne, Niles and Ruth were sitting watching TV. They turned to stare as Julie closed the sitting room door behind us.

"Check it out! Can you believe what Suzy's wearing?" Julie laughed

I wanted so much to leave, to run away, to be anywhere but here but I stood frozen to the spot staring at me black Dr Martens.

"Damn, that's some shirt! Did you actually pay for it?" joked Niles

"At least if you're sick on it no one will notice!" added Yvonne

"Don't think I've ever seen a Hawaiian Goth before!" sniggered Ruth

If it had been a different time and a different place I would have laughed off these comments and thrown in a few juicy self-deprecating ones of my own but as things stood I was feeling incredibly raw and vulnerable and each jibe hit home mercilessly stripping my self esteem and self confidence. I staggered from the room and by the time I had reached the car tears and feelings of misery and self-hatred overwhelmed me.

Sobbing, I drove haphazardly down to the sea front where I parked the car and scraped my knee as I climbed onto the sea wall. It was a blustery day and the wind was merciless and biting. I don't know how long I sat there but I know it was long enough to convince myself not to jump into the raging water. The only thing that ended up in the sea on that chilly February day was my blue Hawaiian shirt.

I recoiled from the idea of bowling and instead retreated miserably to my friend Kim's room in MacIntosh Hall where she patiently listened to my tale of woe and fed me steaming hot cups of tea. I stayed in her soothing presence until late in the evening when I reluctantly decided that it was time to drag myself home.

I had hoped to enter the house and retreat to the sanctuary of my room without meeting anyone but this was not to be; Niles was jogging down the stairs as I carefully closed the front door behind me.

"How'd the bowling go?" he asked

"Uh…fine." I mumbled. Why was I lying?

"Did you play individually or in teams?" said Niles in a valiant attempt at conversation.

"Individually." The pressure of the lie was building up in me and I felt as though it threatened to burst any second.

"So who won?" Niles persevered oblivious to my inner torment.

"Please drop it Niles." I whispered

"Pardon?"

"I DIDN'T GO BOWLING OKAY!" And with that I ran past him up the stairs and shut myself in my room.

God knows what he thought; he was just trying to be nice and make conversation with his rather reclusive flatmate. Unfortunately I was feeling so mixed up and paranoid inside that I was suspicious of his motives and, as a result, frightened to talk and reluctant to explain what had really happened.

That was the term of running away. Even though I had dropped out of Uni my parents and I agreed that it would be better for me to stay in St. Andrews as this was where my friends were and we were satisfied with the medical attention that I was receiving there. The reason I call it "the term of running away" is this: during the week I would spend my time in St. Andrews continually dogged by feelings of depression and despair. I would convince myself that if I returned home to Helensburgh I would leave those bad feelings behind and be okay. So, I would go home and be miserable all weekend where again I would tell myself that if I returned to St. Andrews I would be fine. I was slow to learn that there was no escape from this mental anguish and I desperately tried to convince myself that if only I was physically somewhere else everything would be okay. Who was I kidding? There was no way out of this.

As a means of distraction and a way to supplement my income my parents suggested that I get a job. Yvonne and Ruth had both worked as cleaners in a local Primary school and it was easy for them to arrange an interview for me. I was pleased to be doing something so mundane and requiring so little thought. I was also informed at the interview that I would be working essentially on my own, a factor which pleased me as I had no wish to make conversation with my colleagues. I started my brief employment as a cleaner on a Monday and spent four miserable days on my knees scrubbing floors and cleaning toilets; I immediately became suspicious of my fellow workers and was sure that they were exploiting me and talking about me behind my back. I hated the job so much that I would be overwhelmed with feelings of nausea as I drove my little car to the school. Prior to actually leaving for work I would spend the day shut in my room under the duvet, unable to sleep and battling with torrents of negative thoughts. I was miserable and not for the first time the idea of suicide preyed on my mind. I ended up round at my friend Pete's flat at 2.00am one night depressed and unsure of where to turn. As it transpired I had made the right choice and after a long talk he tucked me into his bed and lay down on the floor beside me so that he wouldn't be far away if I needed him. I quit the job in a characteristically weak and pathetic style: I called in sick on the Friday and simply never went back.

As a more positive means of occupying my time I had started painting and playing the guitar. The paintings were a healthy outlet for the negativity that was consuming me. I would sketch portraits of Batman; a figure whose dark side I could identify with and pictures trying to visually express how I was feeling. One of these paintings showed a character sitting hunched up in a corner as the floor falls away from underneath her. To the side a wall is daubed with words of doubt and confusion and images of fear, pain and darkness.

The guitar playing started because I had swiped my elder brother's battered old acoustic and, armed with a "Teach Yourself Guitar" book proceeded to do exactly that. I have no doubt that Yvonne, Ruth and Niles could have cheerfully strangled me at times as I resolutely strummed away at an E chord, patiently contorting my fingers until they made the correct shape. I didn't like any of the songs in the book so I ignored them and just tried to learn as many chords as I could – practising changing between them as quickly as possible. I was quick to discover that the bad thoughts that plagued me diminished in their intensity whilst I was playing the guitar so I needed no encouragement to practise. Playing the guitar soon became an obsession for me and I continually begged Linda to show me new chords as she was an adept guitar player herself, offering squash lessons in return.

The flat I lived in was never quiet, there were always lots of comings and goings. Linda was pretty much a permanent fixture as she and Niles were an item. One morning Linda's Mum called our house to say that she had just called Linda and Julie's flat but Linda didn't seem to be in which was strange since it was 8.30 am. Where could she be? In a moment of speedy thought and with Linda sitting beside her Yvonne bullshitted that Linda must be on her way round in the car and, in fact, was expected any minute. With that Linda walked to the front door, opened it and rang the doorbell. What do you know; there she was!

"Linda!" shouted Yvonne "Your Mum's on the phone!"

"Toast anyone?" offered Niles as Linda sat down to begin her conversation with her Mum.

I would say that my relationship with my psychiatrist, Dr Paisley, was faltering but for the fact that we had never really bonded in the first place. Whether it was the fact that I was unwell and unable to concentrate or simply just doped up on medication I am unsure, but I was never really able to recall much from our meetings. All I remember is me ceaselessly droning on about how unhappy I was and him altering my medication yet again. If I am to be honest my only real impression of Dr Paisley is of corduroy trousers, a woollen tank top and a beard. I don't say that to be flippant, it is just that he made no particular impression on me and whilst I'm sure he did his utmost to help we just never really connected. I think he realised this too. What I wanted but was scared to ask for was a diagnosis. I wanted a name for why I was feeling the way I felt, to give me some kind of starting point from which to make my recovery. There were times in the middle of the night when I could convince myself that I was going horribly and incurably mad. Surely any diagnosis would be better than that. But I didn't ask. And as a result I didn't get a reply.

The other thing to deteriorate at this time was my friendship with my flatmates – I found it increasingly difficult to talk to them on any level and they, absorbed with their work, made little effort to talk to me. As a result I spent most of my time shut in my room (which I later found out that they misinterpreted as me wanting to shut them out) or round at my friends'. The atmosphere in the flat became extremely tense and I began to believe that they hated me and were happier when I wasn't around. Julie moved in for a brief spell which I was pleased about as I had always enjoyed her company so I was hurt when she made it clear that she didn't want to associate with me either. I desperately wanted to talk with my flatmates and sort things out but I was unable to find either the words or the right time and so nothing was ever resolved.

Although I had left Uni behind for a while I was still involved with the Hockey Club and continued to enjoy playing (unofficially) as a member of the team. My position of choice was goalkeeper and as I strapped on the protective padding and pulled my helmet on over my head I would feel a strength and purposefulness that had long been lacking. As a goalkeeper I was focused and invincible; the "D" around the goal was mine and ultimately I controlled what happened in it. This personality, though one dimensional, was in stark contrast to how I was feeling for most of the rest of the time although ultimately my depression seeped into even this protected corner of my life. I had little concern for my safety – I genuinely didn't care if I got hurt – and this combined with my fast reflexes meant that I was a reasonably adept goalkeeper.

The bond of friendship between the members of the team grew strong as we shared victories and defeats together. I had been playing in the team since first year and as a "second year" was viewed as one of the more established members of the team. I was extremely fortunate to be in a team of tremendous characters; we were there for each other on the hockey field and off and I knew that if I needed help anyone of them would be there for me in a second and likewise. The hockey pitch also provided some much needed moments of humour: my good friend Jane Lloyd was tearing down the wing with the ball kept neatly under her control just ahead of her flying feet when her opposite number, a rather large lady from Fife sporting a rather spectacular pair of cycling shorts, thundered towards her. Jane kept her head and tried to deftly flick the ball past her opponent. Unexpectedly the ball vanished from sight. Everyone stopped. Jane looked round about her and then burst out laughing, pointing at the lady in the cycling shorts – the ball had unfortunately become lodged in the woman's crotch! Luckily, everyone saw the funny side and the game recommenced only to be periodically interrupted by Jane when she collapsed in hysterics as she recalled the incident.

Jane had become a good friend to me over the past months. She had a great sense of humour and wit and was also extremely understanding and a good listener. As a result of our friendship I would spend long periods round at her room in MacIntosh Hall in an attempt to avoid the difficulties in my own house. Jane understood this and gently offered me support and advice as I attempted to sort things out in my head. When I was having a good day my sense of humour would return and we would have some laughs. One time, after an exerting hockey practice, I returned with Jane to her room. I was extremely thirsty and downed a bottle of strawberry milkshake in a "one-er". Shortly afterward, whilst we were chatting, my stomach began to cramp in protest to its milkshake onslaught. I began rolling around the floor in agony cursing strawberry milkshakes and all those who were involved in the production of them from cows through to marketing men. Jane was crying with laughter as she witnessed my moans and contortions and, giggling, encouraged my ranting. Soon the two of us were lying on the floor helplessly laughing and rolling around like hippos in mud. As a result of this I now cannot drink strawberry milkshake or hear its name without a smile being brought to my lips.

The majority of my friends were fantastic during those dark months. I could turn to them for help or sometimes just companionship when I needed it. They continued to include me in their social activities and made it clear that even when I didn't want to be involved I was always welcome. Beth came up for a visit from Manchester (where she had transferred to complete her clinical part of her medical

68

degree). She arrived to find me feeling totally wretched and curled up in a friend's bed depressed and paranoid. We talked for a while, Beth firing off question after question and me trying to get my thoughts together to make reasonable replies – this wasn't easy as I was having one of those days when your brain feels like it's shutting down and getting any sense out of it is a trial. After our talk during which she calmed me down and reassured me, she told me she would be back to see me later and left with a purposeful look in her eyes. I discovered much, much later that she had gone to find Yvonne, Ruth and Niles to express her anger at the way that they were treating me. It wasn't so much that they were saying nasty things, it's just that they gave me no support, didn't try to understand my illness and had made it clear that they didn't want me living with them. To be fair Niles was the only one who made any attempt to be nice.

I was as surprised as anyone when I heard that Beth had given them short shrift; it wasn't my intention that day to put them in the doghouse, I had just been telling Beth what my life was like at that point and I guess it reflected badly on my flatmates.

Of course it could be said that part of the blame for our failing relationships lay with me, I'm the first to admit this, but it would be more accurate to state that the blame should fall at the feet of the illness that I was suffering from. When I'm well I'm a very social and gregarious person but it is the very nature of the condition to be antisocial and as such find it hard to communicate with people. At that point I was having great trouble understanding what was happening to me and because of this, found it extremely difficult to explain how I was feeling to those around me. Out of that group of friends (3rd and 4th years) I found that the only person I could really talk with was Linda. Linda had been going through some difficulties herself and I found that we could empathise with each other, so we would spend long afternoons and evenings sitting by her fire drinking tea and talking about whatever sprang to mind.

Fortunately, however, it was not all doom and gloom. I made some good friends that year, people that I believe I will be friends with for life. I owe a lot to these people, they helped to remind me that there was more to my life than depressive thinking and hallucinations and gently encouraged me to recall my sense of humour and a more positive outlook. I could have quite easily lain in my bed and given up but for the fact that my friends gave me something to look forward to every day. Whether they realise it or not Kim, Pete, Linda, Jane, Michelle, Abby , Jilly, Simon and others played a big part in helping me get through that year. They were there for the good (yes, there were good times!) and the bad as true friends are. I just hope I was there for them as much as they were for me.

One of the problems that I realised that I would have to face whilst writing this is my embarrassingly poor memory. This failing is directly attributed to the medication that I was taking and the side effects that result as a direct consequence. As the year progressed the quantity of medication that I was taking increased and, as a result, so did the side effects. I had the shakes, I felt sick and everything became a blur. I felt increasingly disconnected from reality – as though someone had built a glass wall up around me (although I guess this could be attributed to my illness). My friends commented that I appeared "stoned" a lot of the time and I found taking part in and following conversations increasingly difficult. Although the side effects were wearisome I was willing to put up with them if it meant that my mental health would improve. Unfortunately there was no magic cure and Dr Paisley and I were still looking for the right medication combination for me.

CHAPTER 7

I started back at Uni in the September of 1992 still on medication but feeling positive about my prospects as a student. I had learned some hard lessons the year before and as a result I had decided to return to MacIntosh Hall and take my chances there. I was lucky to be assigned a huge single room on the first floor and spent the first day unpacking, putting up posters and generally making myself feel at home. Later in the afternoon Jane knocked on my door and popped her head round.

"Hiya Stranger! How are you doin'?"

"Jane! I'm good thanks, how are you?"

"Fine. Listen I was wondering if there's any chance that I could tempt you away from the delight that is Hall food and see if you'd like to have dinner at my place this evening?"

"Well I'm not sure" I laughed " it is risotto tonight, you know"

"Mmmm, I see what you mean, rock hard rice was always a favourite of mine too. Shall we see you at 7.00?"

"I'll be there. With bells on. Fancy a cup of tea?"

"Yup, that would be lovely" She paused "do I smell biscuits?"

"Christ, there's no hiding them from you is there. Party rings or choccy fingers?"

"Both. Obviously."

The term began as I hoped it would. I was back enjoying my classes and delighted to be amongst my friends again. During the holidays I had purchased an electric guitar and amp and had brought them to St Andrews with me and I happily thrashed out chords to my heart's content. Whether my neighbours were quite so thrilled I was unsure

73

but I was having a great time! But amongst these welcome good times there was a dark thread that, over time, gradually wound itself tighter and tighter around me. My side effects were becoming increasingly severe and I was finding it harder and harder to cope with everyday tasks and demands. I began to sleep for about 18 hours a day and my concentration dwindled. I felt sick a lot of the time and when I drank alcohol, something I was doing increasingly, I would have huge blackouts.

I was drinking more and more as an attempt to escape from the negativity that was hounding me from the shadows, a means of blocking everything out. It was a frantic, desperate, and ultimately stupid solution that offered more problems than answers but at the time I was desperate for its anaesthetic properties. I just wanted to block everything out. So I drank. For a while everything I did seemed to involve alcohol: playing hockey was an excuse to go to the pub after the match and, likewise, visiting friends was a reason to go and have a drink. I suffered from a particularly vile brand of hangover that develops into a monster as the day progresses and by late afternoon I could usually be found hugging the toilet bowl. Nice.

Alcohol is something that is strongly associated with student life and maybe even without my illness I'd have got myself into trouble. As it was I had enough problems and when news of my drinking filtered back home and I was suffering from increasingly worse hangovers I decided that I had better sort myself out. It wasn't easy. I think like many people the booze is a useful tool if you're feeling shy or unsure in whatever situation – it can help give you the illusion of confidence that is patently lacking. The problem begins when you start to rely on that first, second, third drink to get you through. I didn't yet have a drinking problem but I wasn't stupid enough not to realise that things were heading down a slippery slope and that I had better get my act together. I also realised that I wasn't doing myself or my doctors any favours as my medication became less effective if I was drinking, leaving me wide open to unwelcome symptoms.

I received a surprise visit from Yvonne midway through the term - a surprise because she had won a scholarship to an American college for that year and I recall hiding my pill bottles and telling her everything was hunky dory. I think I felt ashamed of my unstable mood state and erratic behaviour that Yvonne and the others had had to put up with during the previous year and I was desperate to convince her and possibly myself that I had put those times behind me for good.

The following day I was up bright and early in order to make my doctor's appointment at 9:15. As I began the long walk from the Halls to the surgery I reflected on my current situation. My doctor, Dr Boon, had made it clear both to me and my parents that she didn't think that I should return to University as she thought the strain of studying and the student lifestyle was too much for me. After much discussion it was agreed that I <u>could</u> return on the condition that I maintain daily contact with my parents and keep weekly appointments with Dr Boon (as well as continuing to see Dr Paisley). I was, and still am, extremely grateful to my parents for agreeing to this as I feel that returning home to Helensburgh permanently at that time would have been a disaster – I would have lost touch with all my Uni friends and as my Helensburgh friends were all away at Uni themselves I would have been terribly isolated. Besides, I enjoyed my classes and was determined to get a Degree come what may.

As the term progressed, my mood became increasingly erratic – sometimes I would find myself in the depth of despair bleakly questioning the need for my existence and yet at other times I would feel hugely excited and elated. I duly reported these mood changes to my doctors and they responded by increasing my medication again and again until the shelf beside the sink in my room resembled that of a modest pharmacy. So I struggled on with the side effects trying to out sleep the sedation, calm the shakes and I sucked on sweets to help with the dry mouth. But side effects are relentless – they are there when you go to sleep at night and they are there when you wake up in the morning and they gradually grind you down. Keeping your course work up to date whilst all this is going on isn't easy and I was continually frustrated at the standard of my work and my difficulty at making deadlines. I felt as though I was letting myself down. I hadn't realised that this would be so hard.

Dr Paisley had some news for me on my next visit; it transpired that the reason that I was having so many hideous side effects was that I was having a toxic reaction to one of the medications that I was taking. He explained that as a result he would have to gradually reduce my dosage until he could take me off it altogether. Why couldn't I just stop taking it now?

"You have to come off these drugs over time," he replied

I think that was his way of telling me that I was addicted.

By the time the Christmas break came around I was down to about half of the dose that I had previously been taking and I felt that I was doing fairly well. All was fine until just after New Year when my mood plummeted so I made an appointment to go and see Dr Gibson, a local GP. His response once we had talked for a while was that we should immediately return my dosage to its high original level. I explained about the problems that I had been having with the side effects but he argued that his primary concern was to raise my mood from the depths and that we could deal with the side effects later.

I returned to St Andrews for the Spring term on edge and jittery. I was still feeling depressed and my oh so faithful side effects had returned to haunt me. I was coping. I passed my second term exams and handed some essays in. I was getting by. And then, wouldn't you know it, the shit hit the fan.

I had told Dr Paisley about my GP's actions and we had again gradually started to decrease my medication. My mood was still pretty low and I was doing my best to deal with it when I woke from a fitful sleep one morning violently shaking from head to toe. I was feeling very doped but I was alert enough to realise that I was about to be sick and I staggered across the hallway to the toilet. After I had finished vomiting I weaved my way back to my room and passed out on the floor. I was all on my own. To get to a phone would have meant walking along the hall and going downstairs, something I felt completely unable to do. I wrapped myself up in my duvet and stayed on my bed in a semi-conscious stupor interrupted by hallucinations and visits to the toilet. I don't know where the next two days went or what I did but on the third day I finally made it to the phone and called my Mum. Once I had tried to explain what was going on she told me to sit tight and that she would be there in a couple of hours.

She arrived at 4:00 and after she had got me dressed she carefully helped me down to the car and drove me straight up to the doctors' surgery. I was too out of it to be aware of what was going on but I remember that Dr Boon was there to meet us and escorted us into her room. She explained that I would have to come off all my medication with immediate effect and that might mean going through some unpleasant withdrawl symptoms. To be honest I couldn't have given a shit about anything at that moment. She thought it would be a good idea if my Mum stayed for the next couple of days to help me get through the worst of it and she also wanted to see me daily for the next few days.

I'm not sure what was worse: the toxic reaction or the withdrawal. I have a very clear memory of something that happened during that period and I think it sums up how I was feeling. I was in the third day of my withdrawal and even though it was a balmy Spring day I felt terribly cold and tightly wrapped my duffel coat around me. I entered the waiting room to see Dr Boon and made straight for the radiator. I was sweating, shaking and sitting hunched up with stomach pains. There was a young girl, probably about four years old, playing with some toys that were lying around. She smiled at me and I smiled back. Her Mum glanced over, sized me up, and pulled the girl away from me. I felt as if the words "Junkie" were emblazoned across my forehead and I was embarrassed, ashamed and humiliated. I suppose it is something that we all do, judge people by their appearance, but I felt vilified and part of me wanted to go up to that woman and explain my circumstances, tell her that this was not my fault.

Dr Boon suggested that it would be a good idea if Mum took me home for a week or so until the withdrawal symptoms had eased off. I think she also wanted to make sure that I had round the clock supervision as my mood, understandably, wasn't the best. She also explained that such as my situation was at that time she would be unable to put me on any medication to help with my mood swings for the near future as I might react badly to them or, as was the case with the tranquillizers I had previously been prescribed, become addicted to them again. So, wrapped warmly and securely in my faithful duffel coat, I bade farewell to my friends and with my sweaty forehead pressed against the car window whispered a silent goodbye to St Andrews.

I returned after a difficult ten days in good physical shape but shaky mentally. However, it was great to be back amongst my friends again and seeing them did much to raise my spirits and it was good to socialize with them and go out for the odd meal. I think that my biggest problem was that as I was on no medication I was constantly looking over my shoulder waiting for the next episode. I was edgy. I know I should have been "making hay whilst the sun shines" but it was difficult not to be nervous and to think that as I had no chemical defences the next depressive spell might be just around the corner. Happily I made it through to Easter break with no serious mishaps although my mood was pretty low at times. I knew that I had degree exams coming up in May/June and I was already getting pretty worried about them. My concentration was becoming increasingly poor and the big, thick glass wall that surrounded me at times appeared to be returning.

When Summer term came around showing off with its sunshine and beach parties I began to go under. When my psychology tutor, an affable man called Dr Nicols, asked my tutor group to write essays on "Violence" I realised that I was in trouble. The problem was that my brain had stopped functioning on a normal level and I was too distracted with abnormal thoughts to focus on getting an essay written. I went through the motions and took out the relevant books from the library, I even took them back to my room and tried to read them. There was no point. It was as though I had a mental block, I was a terrible person and I should kill myself. That was all there was to it and that was all I could think about.

Part of the problem was that I had lost my objectivity and as such I was not aware that what I was thinking was irrational; when you have delusional thoughts they seem as real as anything that you might have thought before. And, slowly and gleefully, they crucify you. In my own way I was very focused at that time, but unfortunately focused on all the wrong things

There was not a snowball's chance in Hell that I could even begin to write an essay never mind finish one and hand it in. I felt so confused and my brain was like a battleground with thoughts and rationality the casualties. Tears had abandoned me and I felt naked and exposed, vulnerable to any attack. I sat on my bed, books scattered haphazardly on the floor and began banging my head against the wall. The pain and fear that I was feeling was overwhelming and I felt so isolated I couldn't even make contact with myself.

I saw Dr Boon the following day and she strongly recommended that I drop out of Uni once again. She believed that the stress that I was putting myself under was only going to result in more and more serious episodes of ill health. Grudgingly I agreed. I was torn between wanting so desperately to do well at Uni and realising that I was starting to lose control of myself. We agreed that I could stay on in St Andrews until the end of term on the condition that I take next year out to really focus on getting well. The Degree could wait.

I made an appointment to see the Head of the Science Faculty and explained my situation to him. He listened with a grave expression on his face but spoke kind words to me. He explained that what would happen would be that as my course work had been up to scratch I would be placed on a certificate of due performance for the following year. This meant that I would be excused all classes but would be required to sit my degree exams in the Summer. In this way I could take my time regaining my health and sit exams with the minimum of stress.

I spent that Summer making regular trips over to St Andrews to see Dr Paisley. He started me on a new antidepressant which seemed to help a bit but I was still bothered by negative thoughts and suicidal ideation (thoughts and ideas). I also learned to smoke that Summer. It was stupid really; I had just come out of a session with Dr Paisley and I was feeling extremely irritated because I felt that he hadn't really grasped what I was trying to say and I felt that my trip over had been a waste of time. So I was thinking of what I could do that would be both irresponsible and something that he would disapprove of. Alcohol? No, I had to drive home. Drugs? No chance! Cigarettes? Yes, that would do. Stupid, stupid, stupid. So I went and bought a packet of Malboros and drove down to the beach, sat on the dunes and tried to smoke. No one told me how hard it is to light a cigarette from a match when it's windy! Anyway, after much cursing and burnt fingers I finally succeeded in my objective and sat there trying to look cool. The good/bad news is that I wasn't sick and I didn't cough or splutter. I quite liked it. I decided then and there that this would be my secret smoking place and fuck Dr Paisley and everyone else.

I started a brief affair with the Church during the Summer holidays. I have always been quite a religious person; not in the sense that I went to church every Sunday or anything but I have always believed in

God and Jesus. I think I started going to church because I was looking for acceptance and an understanding about what was wrong with me. Unfortunately my timing was off and as I was quite ill that Summer I started to believe that the church members hated me and that God didn't want me in His congregation so I retreated to my bedroom feeling persecuted and alone. My faith has always been important to me but it is a curse of this illness that any type of support, religious or otherwise, will be attacked and warped into something negative, something that will hound and confuse you.

For my fourth year in St Andrews Kim and I rented a lovely little two bedroomed house in a courtyard just off Market street in the centre of town. As ever it was great to be back amongst my friends. Kim had spent the previous year in France and returned full of stories and with a French boyfriend, Phillipe, in tow. Phillipe was lovely, your typical charming, funny Frenchman and he would make various excursions over to France and come back weighed down with wine and camembert.

He also made a little posse of French friends in St Andrews and introduced me to Robert, a handsome French/ Morrocan, who was a very accomplished jazz guitar player. I was smitten and we would spend hours playing the guitar with me trying to convince him that Kurt Cobain was a genius and Robert doing likewise with Wes Montgomery.

I had continued to practise my guitar playing with enthusiasm learning songs and tentatively attempting to make up some of my own. However, I found myself wishing more and more that I was in some sort of band where I could play music with others.

With this in mind I started to let my friends in Glasgow know that I was looking to join a band and, as some of them worked in guitar shops, it wasn't too long before I got a call from a guy who was managing a band that were looking for a rhythm guitarist. So, clutching my guitar I jumped on a bus and headed to Glasgow to meet the band. The band (we never got round to deciding on a name) consisted of a lead guitarist, Jane, a vocalist, Courtney, an amazing bassist, Leo, a succession of drummers and me. We also had a manager, Rick who sported the dodgiest looking peroxide mullet but seemed quite happy with it and no one dared comment. And the music? Well, the music was dreadful. Really. It was kind of a nasty blend of soft rock and cheesy pop but I was so pleased to be in a band that I really didn't mind. Rehearsals were a bit of a joke with everyone else seemingly more interested in getting stoned than practising. Mind you, according to our manager we were destined to be the "next big thing" and I have to thank him for that as if nothing else I learnt a valuable lesson in spotting bullshit at twenty paces. Unsurprisingly, nothing came of the band and when Courtney announced that she was pregnant you could hear the death knell ringing. I was telephoned and told that my guitar playing services were no longer required (I guess my lack of enthusiasm for the music was shining through in my playing) and the last I heard they all went their separate ways the following week.

So I returned to practising in my bedroom determined to improve and equally determined to only play in bands in the future whose music I liked.

CHAPTER 8

I decided that as I wasn't really doing too much with my days other than playing guitar or representing the University at indoor hockey or football I would try and get a part time job. It would have to be something I enjoyed, no school cleaning this time! So I searched through the local paper and visited the job centre finally landing a position as a "School Crossing Patrol Officer" (in other words a lollipop lady!). I enjoyed meeting the school kids and their parents but I was less keen on freezing my ass off outside a school at 8:20am. My friends, however, LOVED it and would take great delight in coming down to the school and taking photos of me in "action".

It was great living with Kim that year. We got along really well and I think I can honestly that not one cross word passed between us. When I was feeling crap Kim would give me space to let me sort my head out, or, alternatively, she would let me know that she was there to talk to if that's what I wanted to do. I was very fortunate and I hope she knows how much I appreciated her.

Our flat, however, had to be one of the coldest places in the northern hemisphere. We had no central heating and I would go to bed wearing thermal underwear, pyjamas, a sweater and a woolly hat plus two duvets on top! It was Baltic! I went through a stage of making myself hot toddies during the day to keep warm when I was studying in the flat. I would have around four or five of them and then be adamant that I was coming down with a bug the next day as I felt so rotten the next morning. I wonder why!

I turned 21 that year. It wasn't the groundbreaking, earth shattering event that I had expected. In fact my 20th birthday was more of a shock; leaving my teens behind was a jarring experience. It wasn't so much that I wasn't ready to grow up and leave my teenage years behind it's just that I seemed to be being forced into it by my age! I remember being given a filofax by my parents on my 20th and being devastated to receive it as I immediately assumed that this was their way of telling me to get a grip and get my life into some sort of order. I hid in the bathroom and cried for an hour cursing myself for not being more successful and capable. Why did I have the problems that I was having? Maybe if I was stronger minded and focussed I would be able to control my health better. Could people do that? I didn't know. I felt pathetic, stupid and well short of my 20 years and I was tired of battling with the negativity that seemed to constantly swirl around in my head. By the time my Mum found me I had convinced myself that I was the biggest loser on the planet and I was in desperate need of her perspective and common sense.

My 21st, however, was a whole different kettle of fish. I counted it as a watershed and I was pleased to have made it that far. There had been times when I was unsure whether I would make it to my 21st but here I was and I was delighted to be. Mum and Dad presented me with a beautiful Fender Stratocaster electric guitar (I think they realised that a string of pearls wouldn't have been the best option!) and then they threw a party for me, inviting lots of good friends and relatives. I had a great day and was thoroughly spoilt by everyone. Party No.2 took place back in St. Andrews where we hired out a restaurant for the night and, aside from a brief altercation when one of my guests took umbrage with a friend of mine because he was gay (twat!), we all spent a very pleasant, if very drunken, evening. The party continued back at my house until the wee hours of the morning, the last of my guests were seen weaving their way down Market street just before dawn.

Dr Paisley and I had reached something of a stalemate and as a result I didn't seem to be making much progress so he suggested that I see a colleague of his, Dr Nicol, over at the Stratheden Hospital. I felt apprehensive about disclosing everything about myself all over again to a complete stranger and from what I recall the visits to Stratheden weren't very productive. Rather than talk to me too much Dr Nicol was keen for me to fill out a multitude of questionnaires which I found slightly irritating as I had studied and torn apart some of these pieces of paper the year before when studying second year psychology. My most memorable encounter at Stratheden wasn't actually with Dr Nicol himself but with a shabbily dressed man who plonked himself down on a seat behind me in the waiting room.

"You a patient then or what?" he asked in a gruff voice.

"I don't know. I suppose. I'm waiting to see Dr Nicol." I replied uneasily.

"No, I mean are you an inpatient?"

"Oh I see. No, I'm just visiting. Are you?"

"Yeah, I am." There was a pause as the man look up and down the corridor. There was no one around.

"You want to get yourself admitted, they've got the best drugs in here." He gave me a sly, conspiratorial grin.

"That's nice." I laughed nervously.

A plump nurse holding a clipboard marched round the corner.

"Suzy Johnston? Dr Nicol is ready for you." She barked.

I turned to say goodbye to my acquaintance but he had gone, melting back into the inner confines of the ageing hospital.

I only saw Dr Nicol a few times after which I was returned to my usual routine of seeing Dr Paisley every fortnight. I still don't know whether the reams of questionnaires that I filled out for Dr Nicol gave any fresh insight into what was wrong with me, maybe they did, but I do know that completing them pissed me off royally and I was glad to be back seeing Dr Paisley.

Robert and I split up amicably after around 3 months and he started seeing another girl pretty soon after. That was fine with me as I was in no real mood to have a boyfriend and it was a relief not to have to appear bright and interesting whenever he was around. It came out in the wash, as all things do, that he had a son back in France. That didn't bother me at all but I was sad that he hadn't felt that he could tell me whilst we were going out.

As luck would have it my older brother, Kit, landed a job working as an assistant manager in one of the restaurants in St Andrews so he came to stay with Kim and myself until he could find himself a place of his own. It was great having him around – he's a pretty easy going guy - although I didn't get to see too much of him as he was working most of the hours that God sends and sleeping the rest.

Summer was coming round and I spent a lot of my time down at the beach smoking cigarettes, playing my guitar and listening to Nirvana albums on my ropey car radio. Kurt Cobain, Nirvana's frontman and songwriter, had stunned the music world by committing suicide in April. Sat alone in his garage apartment overlooking Puget Sound in Seattle he shot up on heroin and placed a shotgun in his mouth. Then he pulled the trigger. The reverberations of that act reached out across the World and touched many people. I was devastated. I had long been a fan of Nirvana's music and I identified with the dark imagery

88

in Kurt's lyrics, his abrasive and yet at times incredibly fragile guitar playing and that voice. That voice. A primal howl of pure emotion that gave life to a rawness of feeling where no words were necessary. I had always kept an eye on Kurt's comings and goings in the music press hoping that he would start to find life less of a struggle. His battle with heroin addiction and intense stomach pains are well documented. But it was his harrowing difficulties with depression that caught my attention. Here was something, and someone, that I could empathise with, someone that I believed could truly understand what I was going through. If I was having a shitty day I would think to myself "Kurt's making it, so can you.". It wasn't much but it helped. So when he killed himself it pulled the rug right out from underneath me. I felt betrayed, angry, sad and yet at the same time I could completely understand why he did it. He had achieved everything he ever wanted and yet still the feelings of self loathing and self hate would not diminish. He had nowhere left to go. But if he couldn't make it what chance did I have? I was scared and quietly mourned a rock star that I had never met.

CHAPTER 9

I needed a job. The Summer job in a guitar shop that I had set up had fallen through and I needed something to occupy me over the Summer break so I was sitting in the library studying and moaning about my luck when one of my friends suggested that I try applying to BUNAC and get a job coaching a sport in America. I applied and was delighted to be accepted and then a few weeks down the line I heard from a Camp, Camp Brentford, telling me that they would like to hire me for the duration of the Summer. Fantastic!

The last few weeks of the term rolled by, punctuated by the two degree exams I had to sit, until finally the last night of term arrived. The Student Union is usually a place of drunkenness and laughter but on this night it was a different story. Dotted around the Bar were 4th year students in tears and the mood was very sombre. People were leaving and it hurts to say goodbye to something that has meant so much over the past four years.

"God, this is depressing," said Micky quietly as he paused to hug another crying student." We can't end the year like this."

"Well what do you propose we do about it?" A stupid thing to say as Mickey was well known for his crazy ideas.

"Yeah, lets do something, something to remember," chipped in Veronica who was standing beside me nursing a very flat whiskey and coke.

"Hmmmm." Thought Mikey "I've got it! It's a warm night, let's go skinny dipping!"

"Yeah!" shouted Veronica "I'm up for it! What about you Suzy? Come on, it'll be a laugh!"

"Oh fucking hell, okay! Don't say I don't give into peer pressure!" I laughed.

We left the depressing confines of the Union still giggling and stopped off at my house to pick up some towels. Kit and Kim were there and we asked them if they would care to join us on our little adventure. Both of them, probably quite sensibly, declined so we grabbed the towels and headed off to Castle Sands beach, a small, secluded cove that joins West Sands with East Sands beach. On the way there the effects of the alcohol I had drunk began to wear off and I started to wonder if this was such a good idea.

"Come on Suzy, it'll be fun – something to really mark the end of the year!" persuaded Veronica.

"Okay, but here's the thing no one, and I mean NO ONE, nicks anyone else's clothes. Deal?" I had heard nightmare stories of people being left stranded on beaches with nothing to wear except a smile. I wasn't amused.

"Yeah, deal. Absolutely," chuckled Micky.

"Sure thing. No stealing of clothes," added Veronica.

We slipped and skidded down the treacherous steps that led to the beach and deliberated on our best plan of attack. Micky pointed to the small wall that acted as the barnacle encrusted boundary between the open sea and the old outdoor swimming pool.

"I reckon our best bet is to run along that wall, dive in off the end and swim for home. What do you think?" he asked

"I guess just paddling is out of the question? Or maybe just easing our way in a step at a time?" I queried.

"Nope. It's got to be diving or jumping in or nothing. It's simply too cold to go in a bit at a time, you'd never make it. No, the only way is to skip along the wall and jump in. It'll take you about thirty seconds to swim back, no problem." Mickey peered at us through the darkness. "Right let's do it. Go!"

And with that he whipped his t-shirt, trousers and boxer shorts off and belted off for the wall, the moon glinting on his naked bottom. Veronica and I looked at each other. "Fuck it!" we both shouted and started tearing our clothes off then we ran for the wall, the cold wet sand squishing between our toes. I hadn't really thought about the coldness aspect of our little adventure but when I counted to three and dived in head first the freezing water seemed to reach up and grab me, enveloping me in its icy grasp. I felt numb. My head was buzzing. I'm not the best swimmer but I swear to

God I could have qualified for the Olympics with the pace that I swam the 50 metres to the shore, leaving Veronica paddling behind me. Then it was out of the water and into the welcoming security of a dry and, in comparison, warm towel. Once we had all dried off and got back into our clothes (Why is it always so difficult to put socks on after you have been swimming?) I felt fantastic. My skin was tingling and I felt healthy and alive. This had been a very good idea and, whilst I would be in no great hurry to repeat it, it rounded off the term beautifully and put some light into what had threatened to become a dark end of term.

My friend Rhona had also become employed by a Camp, through BUNAC, for the Summer and as luck would have it we were on the same flight together. So we both sat back in our seats and toasted St Andrews Women's Hockey Team with Bloody Marys high over the Atlantic Ocean. In fact that whole flight was a bit of a blur as once the air steward discovered we were students he quietly handed over six miniature bottles of vodka and the flight, well, flew by. We arrived in New York and were bussed out to our Camps the following day. I had no idea what to expect. I had heard that the Camps could be quite basic but when I saw the facilities at Camp Brentford I was gobsmacked. There were riding stables, tennis courts, a fully equipped gymnasium, two outdoor swimming pools, basketballs courts, soccer fields, a mini golf course, a base ball field, a nature hut, volleyball courts, a climbing area, a home economics area, art rooms, dance studios, music rooms and ,of course there was the lake. The lake offered all types of water sports from fishing to sailing to water skiing and was in itself an area of calm and natural beauty. The first week at Camp was "kid free" and we were split up into bunks of six with each bunk having at least one returning American counsellor who could answer any questions that we might have. The returning counsellor in my bunk was Debra and she was a great laugh! After we had spent our first day learning about the Camp and playing team building games Debra decided it would be good to take my bunk to Woody's; a nearby bar that was frequented by counsellors. She had also kind of taken me under her wing and wanted to introduce me to Billy, a good friend of her boyfriend Dan. As we entered the bar my eyes began to get used to the dimmed lighting and I saw a good looking guy leaning on the bar. He looked over. Not wanting to stare and feeling a little foolish I let Debra order me a beer. As we drank and talked she mentioned again about Billy and told me to stay put for a bit whilst she went and found him. I stood talking to some of the British girls and felt a tap on my shoulder. I turned round and found myself staring into the brown eyes of the guy that I had seen at the bar!

"This is Billy!" shouted Debra over the noise of the juke box. "You two should talk, I think you'd really get along! Billy, this is Suzy, Suzy, this is Billy. Here are two beers and a table. Get talking!"

Billy and I talked all evening. He was a counsellor at the brother camp of Brentford's, Rockwell, and came from Minnesota where he was at College on a baseball scholarship and he had been hand picked, naturally enough, to teach baseball at Rockwell that Summer. I told him about myself but I was careful not to mention anything about my mental health problems. No one at Brentford knew about them either and I wanted to keep it that way. Anyway, Billy and I were getting along great; he made me laugh and he was a good listener and from the way our hands kept accidentally touching I had hopes that we might be more than just friends.

The first week at Camp was all about getting to know each other and to give the Camp bosses a chance to size us up and to figure out which kids we would be best suited with. After three days I was told that I would be based in the Oaks part of the Camp; the area where the older kids (7th – 10Th grade) would be. I was happy to hear this news as I felt I had more to offer the older kids in terms of guidance and sense of humour and although my teaching duties meant that I would be coaching all age groups, something I was looking forward to, I felt being a counsellor for the older kids would be playing to my strengths.

On the final day of our induction I was told that I would be co-counsellor with Karen and we would be in charge of bunk 22, a 7th grade bunk. In their absence we carefully allotted the kids their beds making sure that the noisy ones were split up and the quiet ones were near a Counsellor in case they felt homesick.

The campers arrived the following day and we were there to welcome them off the school bus that deposited them like many wriggling, excited tadpoles swimming in a sea of shouts and laughter. Armed with a list of bunk 22's names Karen and I hunted down our kids and pointed them in the direction of the bunk where they began jumping on the beds and unpacking their trunks. I couldn't believe it when I looked inside one of those big, bulky trunks; all of the kid's clothes were brand new and still wrapped in plastic bags and each kid had around twenty pairs of trainers: "one for each different activity plus some spares" I was informed.

The next two weeks flew by and I started to get to know my campers and the other kids at the Camp as well. Basically they were all good kids; mischievous, but good fun and kind hearted. The only bunk that seemed to have any problems was bunk 30 where the kids there had decided that they were going to get their counsellors to resign or get fired. Fortunately I had little contact with the girls in that bunk although I felt sorry for their counsellors and counted myself lucky that my campers were such good kids.

Then two things happened that changed everything. The first thing was that I received a phone call from my Mum saying that I had failed my animal physiology and histology degree exam and that I would have to return from Camp early in order to resit it. I was gutted. I was sure that I had done enough to pass that exam and now all my plans of travelling round America after Camp had finished were in tatters. I spent the morning crying on my bed half upset at my ruined plans and letting myself and my parents down, half angry at being so stupid to fail the exam in the first place. I could feel depression tugging on my shoe laces. So I pulled myself together and headed to the Camp hospital and explained to the Head nurse about my situation and past and requested that I be started on the antidepressant that I had brought with me but had had to hand in to the nurses' station when I arrived. The nurse nodded thoughtfully and consulted with the doctor who agreed with me. I was back on the pills after just two months of managing on my own.

The second thing that happened was that Liz, the Head Counsellor, came to find me. She caught up with me after a soccer lesson that I was taking and we sat down on the grass to talk.

"How're things going Suzy? Enjoying it here at Brentford?" she asked

"Yeah, it's great. Hot but great." I joked as I wiped the sweat from my brow – it had been an energetic lesson.

"Let me cut to the chase. We have a problem."

"What's the matter?" I was worried as to how it concerned me.

"First of all it's nothing to do with you. In fact we're very pleased with how you're doing, you seem to fit in very well."

I shrugged. "Thanks; like I said I'm enjoying myself. So what's wrong?"

"We've got a serious problem with bunk 30. One of the counsellors has resigned and we need someone to take her place."

"I see." I could guess where this was going

"We need someone to go in there and take charge. The other counsellor is happy to let the kids get away with anything and they need an authority figure; someone who isn't afraid to be the bad guy if necessary. I'm sure you figured out why I'm speaking to you about this – do you think you could do it?"

"I don't know. I mean I'm flattered you've asked and everything but what about my bunk? I've got attached to those guys and I don't want to just walk out and leave them high and dry." I picked idly at the grass.

"You'll still see them, either in lessons or around the Camp and nothing's stopping you from popping into the bunk to visit them. Plus we've got a replacement counsellor to fill in for you if you decide to take bunk 30 on. Go on. Please?"

"Hmmm. Okay, I'll do it. But I need you to be around to give me support and to back me up if I need it all right? And I want to be the one to tell my own bunk that I'm leaving. I don't want them hearing from anyone else." I looked Liz square in the eye.

"Sure, no problem. Right we'll move you tomorrow. That'll give you this evening to speak to your kids. Thanks Suzy, I appreciate this."

The next morning I pushed open the door to bunk 30 and dumped my rucksack on the floor.

"Hi, I'm your new counsellor!" I shouted above the noise of girls talking and hairdryers.

"FUCK OFF!" they shouted as one and glared at me.

"Okay, we'll try that again; hi, I'm your new counsellor!"

The grumbling response was definitely an improvement and I walked over to my new bed and began unpacking.

I soon realised that if I was to stand any chance of getting them out of bed in time for breakfast I was going to have to make sure that I was up and ready at least half an hour before they were due to get up. And my methods for getting them up? Singing out of tune and at the top of my voice was effective as was dripping water on them, but if all that failed tipping their beds over always worked.

My day as a counsellor at Brentford was exhausting and went pretty much as follows:

7:10 am Wake up, shower and get dressed

7:25 am Wake kids up

8:00 am Breakfast

8:30 am First lesson

9:30 am Second lesson

10:30 am Break

11:00 am Third lesson

12:00 pm Lunch

1:00 pm Fourth lesson

2:00 pm Break

2:30 pm Fifth lesson

3:30 pm Swim time

4:00 pm Shower Hour

5:00 pm Dinner

6:30 pm Evening Activity

8:00 pm Either Evening duty or free time

1:00 am Curfew/ end of Evening duty

1:30 am Go to sleep-dependent on when kids went to sleep. On duty all night in case someone is ill or something is wrong.

One day off a week with two overnight passes over the whole Summer.

Teaching sports all day is pretty tiring but when you take into account the heat that Summer it becomes understandable that most of us ended up in the Camp hospital suffering from heat stroke and exhaustion at least once. To try and combat this I used to run down to the Lake inbetween lessons, strip down to my swimming costume, and jump into the water to try to cool off. By the time I'd got dressed and run back up to the soccer fields I'd have almost dried off.

To keep things interesting all the counsellors taught a number of activities as well as their main one. I taught volleyball, golf, cooking, nature and I worked as a lifeguard (which I loved as I just had to sit in the sun listening to a radio squawk for an hour, signing kids in and out of the Lake area) as well as teaching my chief sport, soccer.

The biggest thing to happen at Camp over the Summer was Leagues. Leagues took place on Sundays and it was when the whole Camp split into two teams, the Americans and the Nationals, and competed in a variety of activities against each other. Leagues usually began at some point in the first four weeks but the actual day and time that Leagues would "break" was kept secret by the Head counsellors. The signal that Leagues was "breaking" was the playing of "Eye of the Tiger" over the tanoy system. The thing is is that it wasn't as simple as that. The previous year a fake murder took place and a "SWAT" team was called in complete with helicopters and as they flew off with the "murderer" in tow, Eye of the Tiger started playing and the kids went mad. This year however a different strategy was planned. Two counsellors, Sally and Dave, pretended to be in love and Dave proposed to Sally at a Camp bonfire in front of the entire Camp. Sally accepted and a few days later they announced that as they had met at Camp they felt it was only appropriate that they should be married at Camp the following weekend and, of course, everybody was invited. So, the following weekend the gymnasium had been transformed into a chapel and the wedding complete with limousines, tuxedos, a wedding dress and a fake minister went ahead. It was only afterwards at the wedding lunch when Dave and Sally took to the floor for their first dance together, after announcing that they had chosen a very special song for the occasion, that Eye of the Tiger started playing and it finally began to dawn on the kids that the wedding wasn't real and that this was Leagues! Crazy behaviour!

Whilst most of the kids at Camp had a great time, some found it difficult. The youngest kid at Camp was just five years old and being away from your parents for eight weeks at age five must have seemed like a lifetime. There was one kid in particular that I kept my eye on, Julie, an 8th grader. I had begun to notice that, after sitting with her at mealtimes for a few days, she wasn't eating. She was also displaying all the classic symptoms of depression – low mood, not wanting to take part in anything, and isolating herself from the other girls at Camp. I empathised with her predicament and really wanted to help so I asked Liz if I could use my free lessons to take Julie under my wing and offer her some one to one contact. After meeting with Liz and the Camp manager to explain the situation and to make sure everything was being done appropriately and with proper supervision I began to meet up with Julie once a day when we went for walks, drank sodas or just watched television. Her mood seemed to pick up but she still refused to eat. Unfortunately I'm no miracle worker and it was eventually decided that it would be best for Julie if her parents came to collect her and took her home. It was a sad day for me when she left and when I think about her I hope her life has got a little easier.

Life in bunk 30 was difficult. It was hard work getting the girls to keep the bunk tidy and to behave themselves around Camp. Fortunately they were blessed with a good sense of humour and we had some laughs but I never bonded with them like I had with my 7th graders and I found myself spending a fair amount of my free time talking to girls and counsellors in other bunks.

My time at Camp was cut short by my requirement to be back in St Andrews studying for and sitting my re-sit exam. Although there were a lot of things about Camp that I loved I was glad to be going home as physically I was knackered and mentally I was beginning to wobble.

I returned to St Andrews and studied hard, sharing a house with my academic daughter, Maisy, where we spent our study breaks lying on our backs in the garden bathed in glorious sunshine staring at the azure sky and smoking cigarettes. I sat, and passed, my exam and was delightfully surprised by my parents when they offered to pay for me to return to America to spend a month travelling up and down the East Coast.

I had a wonderful time visiting New York, Washington, Raleigh, Buffalo, the Niagra Falls and Toronto and was fortunate enough to have a University friend, Scott, living in Manhatten and his parents kindly let me use their apartment as a base. But all good things come to an end and before I knew it it was time to come home and get down to the serious business of completing my final year at St Andrews University.

CHAPTER 10

For my last year in St Andrews I shared a lovely house on South Street with Kim and Abby. Both of them were old friends and I had once spent a very memorable, long, cold walk along West Sands beach with Abby back in second year when it had looked as though we had both screwed up our University careers. That walk and the conversation during it gave us both a speck of hope and helped, in a small way, to turn things around for both of us. From past experience I knew that Kim and I would get on well in our second year of sharing together and I was delighted that Abby had asked the two of us to live with her.

I was slightly surprised when I saw how few courses I was required to take to complete my Degree. One and a half first year courses. Surely that couldn't be right?

I checked with my tutor and he confirmed that this was the case. Fair enough. I was sick of biology and psychology and felt like a change so I picked Moral Philosophy and Ethics, Philosophy of Religion, Logic and Metaphysics and Human Resource Management (I thought it would look good on my CV). I absolutely loved the philosophy classes and Dr Kent, my philosophy tutor, and I hit it off straight away. We had some great discussions during class with me naively offering up basic arguments and she forcing me to question them and come up with better ideas. It was great. Claire and Daniel, two of my classmates, and I would go to the pub after a tutorial and continue our discussions over a pint. I had never felt like this about biology. This is what University was supposed to be about. My only frustration was that I had stumbled across philosophy in my final year and my graduation was fast approaching which spelt the end of my philosophy career, at least at St Andrews.

Management, on the other hand, was a drag. I learned that the previous year the management department had been told to pull its metaphorical socks up as "Too many students were passing" and it was seen by the student body as a "dossy" course. So as luck would have it or rather wouldn't have it they had tightened up and now management was one of the toughest first year courses on the curriculum. I hated it and was soon skipping lectures and blagging my way through tutorials like the experienced fifth year that I was. I managed to get by by forcing myself to read the horrendously dry and dull text that was recommended by the course organisers. It wasn't fun. How people do a Degree in that subject I'll never know.

I was still seeing Dr Paisley and he had added a mood stabiliser to the antidepressant that I had been taking throughout the Summer. He felt that this would even out my moods more as there were times when I felt hugely excitable and on top of the world and then other times when I sank into a dark, broiling cesspool of misery and self loathing. It sounds daft but after seeing Dr Paisley for over three years I had yet to receive a diagnosis. I wanted to know what was wrong with me and I wanted it to have a name. But I didn't ask him. Maybe I was scared of what he'd say. I'd started spending time in the University libraries' psychology section searching for answers to the multitude of questions that I had. I had begun to suspect that I was suffering from manic depression; as well as my tortuous lows I was also experiencing brief spells of mild, but totally inappropriate exhilaration. Highs, for me, were like Christmas Eve at age 4 – a big ball of joy and excitement. My thoughts raced through my head at a

104

thousand miles an hour and I found it impossible to sit still; I even began correcting my tutors in tutorials when I felt they weren't keeping up to speed! Gradually the agitation and high mood would develop into hypomania and I would become irritated at the "slowness" of those around me and find myself singing and laughing out loud for no reason. I'm lucky that this is as far as it went and I didn't become fully blown manic where delusions, hallucinations and destructive behaviour, like emptying your bank account to buy, for example, six cars on a whim become prevalent. Hypomania, or "less than mania" is not so serious but I was quick to learn that a bout of hypomania was often followed by a depressive episode and these I was obviously keen to avoid. Unfortunately whilst I was quick to realise when I was in the grip of a depression I found it hard to identify the highs, as did my friends. I am quite a bright, enthusiastic person by nature and it is only when I became agitated and acted a little inappropriately that my friends and family picked up that something was wrong.

What I read in the library seemed to back up the idea that I might have manic depression but I was the first to admit that I was no doctor and I understood the dangers of self diagnosis so I kept my thoughts and suspicions to myself.

I had another secret that I wasn't ready to share with Dr Paisley or anyone else; a secret that I was ashamed of, a little frightened by and desperate to keep to myself. The previous day had been a bad one; I skipped all of my classes and shut myself away in my room so consumed by fear and misery that I almost felt as though I was about to loose consciousness. Everything felt numb; colours, sounds, everything. I looked around me from my hunched up position on my bed. Chair. Table. Books. Pens. Mathematical compass. I paused then sat up and grabbed the compass. I held the cold, metal object in my hand and then held it against my arm. I stalled again trying to sift through the confusion in my head. I needed some clarity. "How could this help?" I asked myself "how could this help?" I closed my eyes and plunged the sharp end of the compass into my arm. The pain was a revelation; I could feel again, it was sharp, clear and alive, smashing its way through the thick wall of perspex that I had built up around me. The injury was minor; a little blood, nothing that a plaster wouldn't cover up but the feeling of power, the feeling that I could battle the negativity inside me, was enormous. I looked at my arm and smiled when I saw the blood, it proved to me that I was a living breathing Human being and that there was another reality separate from the fog that clouded my thoughts. Liberation. I sat back to think. This had been an unplanned event, if I wanted to do it again I would have to get more organised. Doing it in my room was all wrong – anyone could burst in at any time and a compass? Not very hygienic; I just wanted to hurt myself a little and a visit to the hospital with blood poisoning would attract peoples' attention and that could be very awkward. This was something I intended to keep very much to myself. Razors. That was the obvious weapon of choice and they were openly for sale in any local chemists. I got myself dressed and headed out of the house. It was the first positive thing I had done all day. But there my plan hit a snag. I believed that there were people following me in the town and that others, who might look like normal shoppers to the uneducated eye, were, in fact, spying on me and I felt it was too dangerous to go near the razors in the chemists so I retreated back home frustrated that I had been thwarted. All was not at a loss, however, as I had some cheap plastic razors, the kind that you can pick up at any supermarket, in the bathroom and after examining one quite closely I figured out a way of getting the metal razor out of its blue, plastic casing. Obviously I couldn't leave naked razors lying about in the bathroom so my next thought was where to hide them? I didn't want anyone that might be snooping around in my room to come across them accidentally so I found the perfect place: under the lining of an old jewellery box that I had. I was quite pleased with myself and, as the bathroom had a lock, planned to cut myself in there.

In hindsight, of course, this was a bloody stupid thing to be doing. Self harm is never a solution and can leave the abuser scarred in more ways than one. So what was its appeal? Well, for a kick off, it gave me a feeling of control that I had been lacking for quite a while. I decided when to cut myself, I decided how to do it – this was my choice and it was personal and private to me. It also helped me "feel" when I was depressed and even though all I was feeling was physical pain it still felt like an improvement to the soul destroying numbness that I was otherwise dealing with. Still, these are poor excuses for a violent act and the simple decision to just talk to someone about how I was feeling seems a much more practical and sensible course of action. But things are never that easy. I felt so cut off from everyone that the idea of approaching someone to talk things through seemed almost farcical and when I was ill I wouldn't have been able to maintain a conversation anyway; I was just too scared and miserable so I would turn inward, shut people out and try to deal with things myself. Badly.

I started making myself sick for much the same reasons. Control and self punishment. And a desperation to rid myself of the darkness that so dominated my life. I clutched frantically at anything that I believed that would help me and if that meant making myself vomit then so be it. I tried so hard to cry, many times but the tears just wouldn't come. I felt numb, blank, an emotional mute and I hated myself for it.

So I would sit alone in the bathroom when my flatmates were out and make myself sick and cut myself, pretending to be triumphant but really miserable and unsure of where to turn.

When my mood lifted I was extremely busy. Obviously I had my coursework to keep on top of and there was my involvement as a goalkeeper with both the Womens' Indoor Hockey Team and the Womens' Football Team to keep me active. The thing that I really cherished, though, was the student band that I was delighted to be a member of. The band comprised of myself on lead guitar, Liam on rhythm guitar, Peter on bass, Tom on drums and Shelly on vocals. The band was called "Sub Rosa" and we played mostly covers as well as a couple of songs that I had tentatively penned. It was fantastic for me to hear my little songs played by a full band as I had spent many hours stuck in my room playing the songs to myself trying to imagine what they would sound like with bass, drums and a proper vocalist. Before we knew it we had a gig! It was to be in the Student Union and I remember feeling pretty nervous about it. I had nothing to worry about, however, as the gig went really well and lots of my (drunken) friends came by to watch and cheered loudly. I became good friends with everyone in the band especially Shelly and I would spend most mornings round at her house drinking coffee, playing guitar and smoking fags.

As the first term drew to a close my life was full of contrasts – I was still secretly self harming but doing well academically and on the sports field, sometimes I felt so low that I believe I couldn't have fallen any further and yet at other times I felt invincible. These mood swings were taking their toll and I found that Dr Paisley was keen to increase my medication once again. I complied as I believed the pills to be the only factor that could keep me stable and away from trying anything really stupid.

I sat my end of term exams and waved goodbye to my friends unaware of the opportunity that was about to land at my feet.

I received a phone call from a Tim Grady just before New Year asking me if I would be interested in joining a band as a lead guitarist. When I explained that I was already playing in a band he suggested that I come and meet the "Alkahounds" and make my mind up then. We agreed to meet at Hartly Studios on my birthday, January 4th. Before meeting on that day I phoned round some contacts and asked some questions about Tim Grady. I found out that he was co-manager of Hartly Studios and was managing a promising new band, the Alkahounds. He was reported to be a nice guy and quite trustworthy which allayed any fears I had about him kidnapping me and so I looked forward to our meeting with interest.

January 4th was a cold but dry day and I met Tim at the entrance of Hartly Studios as agreed. He quickly showed me inside and we exchanged some small talk as he led me through the building to the recording studio where the Alkahounds were putting some finishing touches to their demo CD. They were absorbed in what they were doing and didn't hear me enter the impressive mixing room. Tim coughed "Uh guys? This is Suzy-the guitarist that I was telling you about."

I stood nervously looking at the floor eventually raising my head to meet their gaze. There were three of them; Pete, a heavily built man with a goatee in his mid twenties, Rob, a wiry individual also in his mid twenties and Paul, tall and dark haired and probably a little older than the other two. Awkwardly I said "Hi" and commented that, from what I had heard in the past couple of minutes, their demo sounded great. We chatted for a short while about the demo and how it was progressing. I remember that Pete was clutching a Gibson guitar and when he asked me what sort of guitar I had I answered proudly that I was the owner of a Gordon Smith Graduate 60 – the Fender Stratocaster had been traded in a while ago. We seemed to get along well and when Pete asked me if I'd like to come back in a few days to audition I was delighted but a little nervous; I had never auditioned for anything before!

Fortunately the audition went really well and I was pleased to discover that Pete and I shared a common interest in a lot of bands and seemed to be coming from the same place when it came to making up songs. I spent the next few days practising with him and learning the required parts and by the time it came for me to return to Uni I was a fully fledged Alkahound and I would spend the rest of the academic year travelling between St Andrews and Glasgow to make rehearsals.

I arrived back at University thrilled to be in the band and no doubt bored a few friends rigid by playing them the demo over and over! However, my enthusiasm for my own band in St Andrews hadn't diminished and I was more determined than ever to write more songs and get more gigs.

This was to be a busy term for me and once again I was struggling mentally. I was trying so hard to hide how I was feeling from everyone, especially my new bandmates and new boyfriend Will. I had known Will for years and we had started going out after a cunning plot by friends who thought we'd go well together. Our first night together, however, had been a disaster. I had my period and was suffering from excruciating period pains and, once Will had gone to sleep, had crept down to the toilet where I spent the rest of the night throwing up and writhing in agony. When Will woke up in the morning he took my absence to mean that I didn't like him and was trying to avoid him. Nothing could have been further from the truth I just thought that I would spare him the grimmer side of my menstrual cycle!

I realise now that I should have at least tried to explain to Will how I was feeling rather than just assuming that he wouldn't understand but I guess I was too frightened that I might lose him. Of course shutting someone out is not conducive to a good relationship and ultimately, even at the beginning, spelt the end for Will and me.

My cutting spells increased as my mood deteriorated and I was finding it harder to come up with excuses that covered the multitude of scratches and cuts that appeared on my arms and hands. Maybe I wanted to be caught. Maybe I wanted someone to realise how difficult I was finding life at that time and to magically sort things out for me. My mood was reflecting in my work as well. I was called to meet with Dr Kent, my philosophy tutor, after writing two essays; one defending the right to commit suicide and the other examining the possibilities of life after death. In the confines of Dr Kent's smoky office I did my best to explain how I was feeling at that time but as I said them the words sounded clichéd and tired and I was once again disgusted at my inability to articulate my thoughts. One thing that I did manage to get across, however, was that I would be unable to sit the end of term exam as I simply wasn't able to study and retain any sort of relevant information. Luckily Dr Kent was a kindly individual who realised my plight and agreed that it would be futile for me to sit any type of exam, instead suggesting that I write another essay in my own time and that they would use the mark from it as my exam mark. If I had been able to cry I would have; I was extremely grateful. I have no doubt that if she hadn't suggested this I wouldn't have graduated that year.

I continued to play sport and found that concentrating on a hockey game or a football match helped distract me a little from the depression that was swarming around me. We had surprised everyone, including ourselves, by winning the Scottish Universities' Indoor Hockey Championship and as a result found ourselves on a coach heading down to Bath to represent the Scottish Universities in the British Universities' Tournament. Ours was a team in the truest sense of the word; none of us were internationals and yet we played together with a fluency and anticipation that would have made you think otherwise. The key to our team was that we genuinely liked each other and knew each others games so well that we could easily predict everyone's moves and passes during a match.

The Scottish Universities Tournament in Edinburgh had been a riot; our hockey had been sensational and our supporters were warned with eviction for being too loud! We carved our way through the opposition and defeated favourites Herriot Watt convincingly in the final – this was quite an achievement as the Herriot Watt side was made up mostly of internationalists and had a reputation for not giving much away. We celebrated by driving through the streets of Edinburgh holding the trophy high through the sunroof of my car. The irony of the situation for me was that I had got through the whole tournament without so much as injuring a finger and yet managed to damage my right knee when I fell on a rock during a drunken game of Kamikazi – running blindfolded through the sand dunes at West Sands beach; last one left standing wins – at a party that night back in St Andrews. Fortunately I was fully recovered for our trip down to Bath and I couldn't wait to see how we'd fare against the best in the country.

The whole adventure down South nearly came to a catastrophic end when our coach blew out its two left rear tyres on the motorway and we skidded to a halt. God; I owe you one. Thankfully our driver, Red, was a fully paid up AA member and we didn't have to wait too long before we were up and running again. However, because there had been a delay we were running a little late and, in order to make it to our first game in time we (no doubt to the delight of the passing commuters) had to change on the bus.

I think the thing that surprised most of us when we finally arrived at the tournament was how professional everyone looked. Each team had Managers, Physios, Coaches, a multitude of substitutes and matching tracksuits. We had matching kits and three substitutes. No Coach, Manager or Physio, just us. We realised immediately that we were viewed as the underdogs and we rallied to the challenge finishing top of our group and lined up to play Loughborough, the top P.E. university in the UK, in the semi finals.

By the time the Loughborough match came round we were all knackered and injured in some way or another and as we had so few substitutes we weren't afforded the luxury of being able to rest players. We didn't really think we could win, I mean this was Loughborough for goodness sake, but we decided to give the game our all and see what happened. The teams that had been eliminated from the tournament had stayed on to watch and by now we had quite a group of supporters backing us which egged us on. At half time the score was 1-1 and everything was going well apart from one thing. When Loughborough scored, their centre forward collided with me as she pushed the ball into the back of the net. Her right knee had smacked into my left temple which had left me feeling groggy and with double vision. Jane, our captain, and Rhona took me aside and tried to suss out whether I could continue. I was adamant that I was staying in the game and brushed off any concerns that they might have about concussion. I was fine. To be honest I don't remember much of the second half but I do know that we all played out of our skins and Jane scored a beautiful goal to give us a famous 2-1 victory over the mighty Loughborough and set us up for a rematch against Durham in the final!

I only managed to play the first half of the final as I was feeling too damn nauseous to stay on the pitch and, unfortunately, the game was lost by then anyway. If we had had more substitutes then maybe we would have stood a chance, after all we had drawn with Durham earlier in the tournament, but as it was we were all too tired and sore after the Loughborough match to put up much of a fight and we ran out 7-1 losers. I didn't hear of the final score until much later as I was bundled into the back of Jane's Mum's car and driven to Bath's Accident and Emergency Dept with a suspected concussion. After a short wait I was shown through to a cubicle where I gratefully lay down on a bed where I was asked a whole host of questions and examined by a young, white coated doctor, Dr Nash. Dr Nash poked and prodded me which I put up with without complaint until he mentioned that he needed to look at my feet and could I take my trainers off? Embarrassed, I warned him that as I had been playing hockey all day my feet probably didn't smell too good! After he had finished with me and my smelly feet he left the cubicle for about thirty minutes during which all of the members of the hockey team popped in to visit and to steal something as a souvenir. Laughing that they were going to get me arrested I kicked them out and when Dr Nash returned only Jane and her Mum remained. He explained that they wanted to keep me in, at least overnight, as I had a concussion and they were slightly concerned about the double vision I was having. When I asked what was causing it he said that where I had been hit on the head had probably caused some bleeding in my left eye socket which would account for the double vision. Oh. I thanked Jane's Mum for her care and the trip in the car to Casualty and asked Jane to come and pick me up at breakfast the next day as I was determined to travel home in the coach with the team.

After everyone had left and I had been given something to deaden the throbbing headache that was pounding in my head, I was plonked in a wheelchair and pushed through the sunny, light corridors of the hospital which echoed with the voices of busy doctors and nurses. I was finally pushed into a two bedded room which was already occupied by another female patient with black hair and aged about forty.

"This is your bed Suzy, get changed into that robe and I'll be back in about thirty minutes to check on you both. Oh yeah, this is Angela, she'll keep you company." Commented the nurse who had had the joy of wheeling me through the hospital.

"Uh nurse? Could I have a shower first? I've been playing hockey and I'm sure I don't smell that great" I asked.

"Wait until I come back okay? We don't want you keeling over in the shower now do we?"

"Okay."

The nurse left the room and as I sat down on the bed I glanced shyly over at Angela.

"Hi, I'm Suzy. How're you doing?"

"Okay. Thumping headache but okay. Could murder a fag though, do you smoke?"

"Yeah I do but I don't think smoking's allowed in hospitals. Something to do with it being unhealthy or so I've heard."

"Ha ha, I know what you mean. They'd be in here like a flash if they smelled the smoke."

I paused and looked at the window.

"You know, if we could get that window open we could probably smoke a cigarette out the window and they'd never know. What do you think? Will you give me a hand?" I asked as I walked over towards the window.

Angela joined me and together we heaved at the ancient window frame. Suddenly with a rush and a blast of cold, fresh air it was open and Angela pulled out a crumpled cigarette packet. I took a fag from her and lit it, inhaling deeply.

"Aaah, that's better! So, Angela, what are you in here for?" I queried.

"Concussion. How about you?" She replied dragging on her cigarette.

"The same. I got whacked on the head playing hockey. I'm the goalie." I explained "How about you? How did you end up with your concussion?" I asked.

"I...no, I can't tell you it's too embarrassing."

"C'mon it can't be that bad."

"No, really, it is"

My curiosity was piqued, what could have happened to her?

"Angela look, I'm a complete stranger and tomorrow, God willing, I'm heading back to Scotland where you'll never see me again. What's the harm in telling me?" I stubbed my cigarette out and flicked the butt out of the window.

"Okay. Well, you see I had decided that I was going to cook a leg of lamb for my husband's dinner."

"Uh huh."

"So I went over to the freezer – we have one of those low, horizontal freezers where you have to lift the lid up – and lifted out the frozen leg of lamb. But the thing was there were some sausages stuck to the leg and I couldn't prise them off. I tried with my fingers and then with a knife but it was no good, those bloody sausages wouldn't move." She paused and shifted from one foot to another.

"C'mon Angela! Don't stop now! What happened next?" I urged her on.

"Well...I got so angry with those damn sausages that I picked up the leg of lamb and smashed it down on the lid of the freezer. I didn't expect the rebound and it caught me square on the forehead! I lay there, unconscious with the lamb slowly defrosting, until my husband came home and found me." She looked quite forlorn.

"Oh Angela, that's marvellous!" I hooted "That's the best reason for a concussion that I have EVER heard. Fantastic! You should be proud of it!"

"Really? You don't think it's stupid?" She smiled a little half smile.

"No way! It's genius! Think about it, you must see how funny it is." I wiped the tears from my eyes.

"Heh, heh, yeah I suppose it's pretty funny."

By the time the nurse came back in the two of us were stood by the opened window howling with laughter. It was the first time I had really laughed hard for ages and it was a relief to know that I still could.

The following morning, after having spent a delightful night being woken up every hour to have a light shone in my eyes, I said goodbye to Angela and discharged myself. Jane and Simone picked me up at 8.00am and we headed back to Simone's parents' house where the bus was waiting to return us to St Andrews.

CHAPTER 11

I continued to rehearse with the Alkahounds and played my first gig with them at the 13th Note, a small club in Glasgow. I was terribly nervous and didn't play particularly well but I was glad to get the gig under my belt. We played a few more shows soon afterwards and with growing confidence I suggested that we play a gig in St Andrews. The boys thought that that would be a great idea so I arranged a gig in the Student Union with Sub Rosa supporting. The gig, otherwise known as "Suzy showing off that she can play guitar night" went really well and Pete sang guest backing vocals on a couple of Sub Rosa songs which was great. However, I was still unhappy with my performance and vowed to practise more and more until I had ironed out the faults in my playing. I was starting to feel concerned that I would be fired from the band if things didn't suddenly and dramatically improve and this added pressure didn't help my mood. We played another gig at the superbly named King Tut's Wah Wah Hut in Glasgow and although I felt that I played better I could sense that Tim wasn't happy with my performance. Pete had become a good friend in the short time that I had known him and it was him that I turned to with my worries and concerns. He reassured me that I was not going to be kicked out of the band. We began spending a lot more time together writing songs and just hanging out as friends. My influences and style of guitar playing brought a harder edge to the band and Pete seemed to embrace this and was pleased with my contributions. It was good to be around him and I felt relaxed and comfortable in his presence. I talked to him openly about my mental health problems and he was sensible and reassuring in his response. He was a good friend but for me it was never going to be more than that. So when he started sending me poems and clever, little word puzzles I should have been more astute and handled the situation better and nipped it in the bud. But I didn't; I suppose I was flattered and didn't want to hurt his feelings. Maybe I thought that eventually I might fall in love with him but I soon realised that these things can't be forced or happen just because you care for someone as a friend. Things came to a head one night when the two of us were sitting in my car after a rehearsal. He told me that he loved me and he wanted to know how I felt about him. Weakly I told him that I really cared about him but I wasn't in love with him and that I couldn't see our relationship as it was progressing any further. I was sorry. I don't think I could have hurt the poor guy more if I had punched him in the face. Holding back tears he told me that I would change my mind and clambered out of the car.

Things changed after that night. I had secured my place in the band but I had lost Pete for good. He would blank me when I tried to talk to him only replying when the question was something technical about a song and you could cut the atmosphere at rehearsals with a knife. He seemed to hate me and could hardly bear to be in the same room as me. I was miserable and would often slip into depressive reveries during rehearsals, finding it easier to disappear inside myself than to face and deal with the torrid emotions in the room. Incredibly Rob and Paul seemed to be oblivious to the unhappy vibe and cheerfully carried on playing the songs without noticing the difficulties that Pete and I were having. The song writing process became very awkward as it required Pete and me to be together in the same room on our own without the ice breaking qualities of either

120

Rob or Paul. In retrospect I think we only managed it because we put the songs to the forefront and focussed on them. But it wasn't fun. The only reason I stayed in the band was because I believed that our music was good enough to go places and I was fiercely proud of our songs and everything that we had and, hopefully, were going to achieve. Plus I hoped that someday, somehow Pete and I might become friends again. I missed him.

Summer term came round and I paused when it hit me that this would be my final term at St Andrews. Those five years seemed to have flown by and soon, after eighteen years of educational padding, I would be forced to find my way in the "real" World and discover my place. A daunting prospect. Happily though I still had one more term to enjoy and I was determined to make the most of it.

I received news in April that I had been selected to represent the Sottish Universities at football. I was thrilled and even more delighted when I was informed by the Coach that I was to captain the team in our annual fixture against England. We lost a good hearted game in Newcastle by 2-4 and, although I didn't play particularly well, we all enjoyed the occasion. As a direct follow on from that I was honoured to be awarded a "Blue" - the highest sporting award - by the University which now hangs with pride on a wall in my parents' house.

I had two exams to sit that term – one in Logic and Metaphysics and one in the dreaded Management. The Metaphysics exam was only an hour long and I sat it in a Hawaiian style outfit. The reason for this will become clear. I answered a question on the Theory of Infinity which took about fifteen minutes to write and then I lent back in my chair revelling in the feeling that this was my last ever exam. I emerged from the exam hall at the end of the exam and was immediately covered in powdered milk, rotten eggs and fizzy wine as my friends celebrated the completion of my last "Final" in the traditional manner. Then it was off to the pub, still covered in all this crap, to, again as tradition states, down a shot. All I remember is hurriedly drinking some whisky before being evicted from the pub because I smelt so bad!

The Management was a different kettle of fish and I struggled manfully to answer the required questions: I didn't like the subject and it was fairly apparent that the subject didn't like me. I waited nervously for the results only to be informed that as the Management scores were so bad – the word was that over half of the candidates had failed – that the results wouldn't be posted on the notice board as usual. Instead we had to go and individually pick up our marks from the head of the department. Lovely.

I took a deep breath as I stood outside the Head of the Management Department's office, nervously knocked on the white, wooden door and, offering a silent prayer, crossed my fingers and toes.

"Come in!" barked a voice that didn't sound as though it was used to being kept waiting.

Gingerly I pushed the heavy door open and carefully closed it behind me.

"Uh, hi. I've come for my first year exam result."

"I see. Name?"

"Suzanne Johnston"

He pulled out a wad of paper and began to flick through it. My eye briefly caught names and numbers printed beside them. Most of them seemed to be under 50%.

"Ah yes. Suzanne Johnston. 56% young lady, you should have done better you know."

Relief flooded over me like a warm, soothing liquid. I had passed. I had passed! I tried my best to keep the idiotic grin off my face until I exited the Management Department for the last time and let loose my exuberance by jumping up and down in the car park secure in the knowledge that as I had already picked up 75% in Metaphysics I would definitely be graduating that Summer.

The magnitude of the event of me finally achieving my goal of gaining a Degree didn't hit home until much later. Mine had not been the smooth trip through University that is boasted about in the prospectus. I had struggled and crawled, losing my way many times and when it came to strength, courage and faith this Degree was as much my parents and friends as it was mine. These had been five of the most wonderful and terrible years of my life. Of course I had learned a multitude of facts and figures but these seemed to pale in comparison to hard lessons that life had thrown at me and the fantastic friendships that I had made. I owe a huge amount to my parents and their belief in and understanding of me. They realised, probably more than I did at the time, what the cost to me emotionally would have been if I had not stayed in St Andrews and had the chance of completing my studies and staying in the close proximity of my friends. It would be wonderful to be able to say that as I left University behind so my mental health problems dissipated but University had never been the major problem, I had, and escaping from myself proved to be a difficult task.

CHAPTER 12

Graduation was a sombre, grand and hilarious occasion. The actual ceremony for the degrees of Bachelor of Science's took place in Younger Hall on a sunny Wednesday afternoon and I remember that I was dreadfully hungover. My friends and I had arrived in St Andrews the previous afternoon and spent the evening in the pub getting extremely drunk . I woke up the next morning with a throbbing head and the desire to stay in the vicinity of a toilet for at least the immediate future. My parents arrived bright and perky soon after I had struggled out of my bed and changed into my clothes. We had arranged to meet Kim and Abby and their respective parents for lunch in a small nearby town, Elie. What my parents had forgotten to mention was that the restaurant that we would be dining in was a fish restaurant and the fishy wafts from the kitchen drove my already nauseous stomach into overtime. We were seated and I scanned the menu whilst maintaining an admirable, under the circumstances, amount of small talk with Abby's and Kim's parents. I decided the safest option for me was to order the only non fishy item on the menu which happened to be the all day breakfast. When it arrived I was halfway through my second sausage when I realised that I was about to be sick. Hurriedly, I made my excuses and, with Abby and Kim offering gentle applause, rushed to the restaurant's rather plush bathroom where I was reacquainted with my lunch. Shakily, I returned to the table where I was greeted by sly smiles from my flatmates and concerned looks from my parents.

After lunch my parents and I went for a long, brisk walk along the beach at Elie and the fresh air proved to be a wonderful tonic and allayed any fears that I had had about being the first student in the history of St Andrews' University to puke during the Graduation ceremony.

We returned to St Andrews and spent a lovely hour taking in the sights, sights that I had taken so much for granted over the past five years, and I said some quiet and personal farewells to the grand buildings that housed my studies as a student. Our final destination was Younger Hall where the Graduation ceremony was to take place. I picked up my gown and my brightly coloured cerise hood with white fur edging (I had always thought that the Divinity student's purple and white hood was far more attractive!) and paid close attention when we were directed as to how the actual process of graduating proceeded. According to tradition we had to individually step onto the stage and wait until our name was called. Then, holding your hood, you walked up to the Dean of the University and handed your hood to the man standing on the right and kneel down. You were then patted on the head by a piece of John Knox's breeches and had some Latin said over you. As this was happening your hood was placed over you and when this was done you stood up, took a step back and bowed to the Dean. Then you were given your scroll and could return to your seat. Phew! All of us were terrified that we would, in some way, mess it up and make complete idiots of ourselves. My biggest concern, however, was that my gown was too long for me and I was worried that as I stood up after kneeling I would step on my gown and go flying backwards off the back of the stage! That would be something for my Dad's video recorder! Fortunately, everything went smoothly and I found myself both moved and extremely proud of the pomp, tradition and ceremony of

126

the occasion. It was a fantastic way to end my University career and will always be engraved on my memory.

Summer arrived and with it came the opportunity to take a course to upgrade my Scottish Football Association C licence to a B licence. I arrived on the course feeling nervous and more then a little out of place; I was the only female taking the course. Fortunately, however, the guys on the course, all either professional players or coaches, made me feel welcome and were quick to include me in the banter that was flying around. I was particularly looking forward to the goalkeeping aspect of the course and relished the opportunity of meeting and talking to Alan Hodgekinson, the Scotland goalkeeping coach. I was to be sorely disappointed. Time and time again I volunteered to take part in one of the goalkeeping exercises that were being demonstrated and time and time again I was ignored. My blood was boiling. Eventually, the final exercise came round, involving shots on goal from various angles, and I could stand it no more. I stood up, walked over to Alan, grabbed the goalie gloves off him and said "I gather it's my turn now."

There was no way on earth that I was going to let any of those shots get past me, even if it killed me! I saved everything and rounded off my "clean sheet" with a spectacular, acrobatic, diving save to the top, right corner denying former internationalist Alan McInally a goal. That save left me with a badly staved thumb (he hit the ball so damn hard) but I didn't flicker and defiantly handed the gloves back to Mr Hodgekinson. All the guys broke into spontaneous applause with one bloke, Andrew, leaning close to me and laughingly whispering "You're a bloody show off Johnston!" Before I headed off to get my thumb looked at I was hoping for the chance to have a chat with Alan but he made it clear he wasn't interested in speaking to me and I was left disappointed and angry. Unfortunately this was the attitude of most of the SFA coaches in charge of the course; they just didn't seem to want me there because I was female, an attitude I found frustrating and downright offensive. I felt I was being undermined in everything I did whether it was on the football field or in the classroom and unsurprisingly I failed the course. The saddest thing about the whole situation is that it has put me off attending any more SFA courses and ultimately put a damper on any interest that I had in football coaching.

I found it difficult readjusting to life back at home on a permanent basis and away from my University friends. Most of my Helensburgh friends had gained employment away from home and so I was left feeling pretty isolated and alone. Depression lurked. I felt useless and surplus to requirements and although my parents seemed happy to have me back at home I felt as though I was constantly under their feet and was frustrated at my financial inability to move out. The darkness began seeping its way back into my life and I felt apathetic and miserable. There were plenty of people on hand to offer advice and I nodded sagely and agreed to everything they said as it seemed easier than offering any resistance. I hated myself and the negative emotion built up in me like a putrid abscess. For so long my focus had been achieving a Degree but now that I had done that I was adrift and goalless. I had put a lot of thought into what I was going to do with my life and unfortunately I was the first to admit that a big city job was not for me as, like many people, I didn't feel that I would cope at all well with the stress that seems mandatory with that sort of employment. So I looked at the alternatives and decided that primary school teaching seemed like the most attractive option. But I had no experience and, as I realised that primary teaching was a very popular choice for a lot of graduating students, I decided that I would approach my former headmaster and ask his advice. He was very helpful and suggested that I work as a volunteer in the school's primary department and also work as a tutor in the girl's boarding house, Lansdowne.

Still sludging through the mire of depression I painted an acceptable smile on my face and began working at the school. I soon found, however, that I enjoyed working in the primary department, especially primary one where I would help a boy who was lagging behind his classmates. It was fun and, luckily, I seemed to be good at it. I really began to believe that I had made the right decision and that teaching would be right for me.

Being a tutor in Lansdowne was fairly straightforward and enjoyable. I was on duty one day a week and the occasional weekend. The girls in the house were great and lots of fun to work with and, barring a few incidents when people misbehaved or when I had to play "good cop/bad cop" with the Housemaster when I caught some juniors smoking, everything went fairly smoothly. I respected the girls and they respected me. They knew that I was happy to have some fun and a laugh but I would only let myself be pushed so far and that rules were rules. The other tutors were, on the whole, good people and easy to get along with. The girls heard me playing my guitar in my room in the house and were curious about it. I told them about the Alkahounds and made a mental note to organise a supervised visit to one of my all ages gigs.

Depression continued to slouch through my veins and although I feel that I successfully hid it from most people it was my GP, Dr French, who received the brunt of it during my once weekly visits. I would open up and talk about how I was really feeling deep down inside, in that place that I kept hidden from everyone else. God, how I moaned! But I realised that I needed to offload how I was feeling to someone and the years of seeing Dr Paisley had made me realise how important talking can be and I greatly appreciated Dr French for being there to listen to me. She responded to my tales of trauma by changing my antidepressant to a newer model and told me to persevere with it. Unfortunately I found the side effects unbearable; I felt terribly sick, had the shakes and had to wear dark glasses all the time as my pupils were constantly dilated and, as a result, I found any sort of bright light extremely painful. I went back to see Dr French after a week and she agreed that the best course of action would be for me to return me to my original antidepressant.

I began to spend most of my free time at home and away from the isolation of my room in the boarding house. I knew this move wasn't popular with the Housemaster and Housemistress, the MacKays, but I couldn't help it; I needed to be around my family as I found that spending time alone in Lansdowne gave me too much time to think and caused my bad thoughts to run haywire. I found that as my mood sank I was becoming increasingly preoccupied with thoughts of suicide and death. I would become obsessed with ways of planning my demise and spend morbid hours counting my pills and wondering how many I would have to take for it to be fatal. I didn't act on any of these thoughts but it was a distressing place to be. However, at the same time I found the idea of committing suicide strangely tempting and the idea that, if the mood took me, I could do it bizarrely comforting. This was my secret and was, like self harming, something that I could control. So I would plan in minute detail how I would do it and analyse the pros and cons of hanging, overdose, jumping from the roof, or slitting my wrists. I was so engrossed with these thoughts that I found it hard to spare any consideration for my family and the ones that I would leave behind. I was totally selfish and unable to see the bigger picture. Don't get me wrong; I loved my family: it's just that I was so unhappy and thought myself so worthless that I simply didn't appreciate that they would miss me. I wouldn't have missed me. Eventually I began to talk to Dr French about these feelings and, after some careful questioning, I think she believed me when I promised that nothing would happen. Nothing did but it didn't stop the thoughts from spinning around in my head. The darkness inside me felt palpable and I believed that if someone were to cut me open they would find a black, oily liquid oozing through my body. I was consumed by it and the medication didn't seem to be helping.

Dr French left Helensburgh after her rotation was up and I felt abandoned and discarded. This was someone that I had really opened up to and now that she had left I felt back at square one and I didn't know where to turn. However, all was not lost, Dr French had left recommending that I see a Community Psychiatric Nurse, Shiela Brackett as an alternative. Unfortunately, it wasn't to work out. Shiela arrived dressed totally in black and her manner did not inspire optimism. Mostly, however, I was irritated by her habit of picking words out of my sentences regardless of context and focussing on them. I hadn't got the measure of her at that time and I knew it was extremely unlikely that I was going to open up to her at least until I was sure I could trust her. It was obvious that she had been primed by Dr French about my suicidal ideation, and rightly so, but it was all she wanted to talk about and I felt uncomfortable and ill at ease. In retrospect she was acting completely appropriately but I think I would have found it easier if we had broken the ice first by talking about something a little more lightweight. I tried answering her questions but it felt awkward and unnatural and everything that came out of my mouth sounded all wrong and every bone in my body screamed "Watch out!". I wanted her to leave and when she did I knew I wouldn't be seeing her again.

CHAPTER 13

My mood picked up a little over Christmas which was fortunate as I had an interview at Jordanhill College of Education to deal with. The interview consisted of a group debate, a written essay and an interview by a panel. The group debate went well; it was a debate about the prison service and I was careful to be neither too dominant nor too passive but made sure I took an active part. I also felt that the interview itself was fine and I received positive responses from each of the interviewers and we talked at great length about my experiences in America which they seemed extremely interested in. Finally, the written essay. What a disaster! I didn't have the first clue about the question which was about the nursery school voucher system so I mentally rolled my sleeves up and made a brave attempt at bullshitting my way through it! I have no idea what the person that read it thought but it must have been okay as I was delighted to be given a place in the next academic year's roll.

Jordanhill is an unfortunately ugly Campus. It is made up of a myriad of grey modernistic buildings and the dark oppressive skies of that chilly September day did nothing to detract from the depressive atmosphere. But I hardly noticed, I was too excited to be beginning my course and looking forward to meeting my classmates so I walked with a spring in my step and entered the front door. To the right of the main entrance was the cafeteria and loads of people were milling around inside. I paused and, feeling a little nervous, went in and immediately became overwhelmed in a sea of unfamiliar faces. I joined the human snake that coiled its way to the canteen servery and, fumbling in my jean pocket for some change, tripped and bumped into the girl who was standing in the queue in front of me. I apologised and we began chatting aided in no small way by the fact that both of us were feeling a little anxious and had yet to exchange a word with anyone else that morning. Her name was Rita and although it turned out that she was in a different class from me we were to become good friends and I would spend many evenings round at her flat drinking extremely strong coffee.

At 9:00am the cafeteria was deserted as everyone rushed off to their classes and I became anonymous in the crush heading off to primary education. The morning was spent "getting to know each other" and taking part in team building exercises which were fun and involved the building of towers out of paper, plastic straws and sellotape. Blue Peter would have been proud. Then we were called individually to see the Campus doctor for a brief medical. Immediately my alarm bells started ringing. I had neglected to mention in either my application form or interview that I had any mental health problems, mental health problems that had only recently been confirmed as manic depression. Shit. When it was my turn to see the doctor I questioned him quite carefully about his confidentiality policy and only once he had reassured me that no one on the course would be privy to any information that I might share with him did I relax and tell him about the problems that I had been having. He was curious but assured me that as long I was having adequate support at home and that I came to see him once a term he had no problems with me continuing my studies at Jordanhill. Maybe I was being paranoid but I had decided long ago that no one connected with my course would find out about my illness: the words "manic depression" and "primary school teacher" just didn't seem to sit too well together. I knew that, of course, I wasn't a danger to anyone but I also appreciated the stigma that surrounds mental illness and the last thing I wanted was to become a victim of it. So I played my cards close to my chest and made another mental note to myself to be very careful whom I shared that information with.

After a few hypo manic days where I had been zooming around the Campus and at the centre of every conversation and classroom discussion, even summing up for and correcting our tutor when I felt he wasn't making a good enough job of it, the dark clouds, like those looming over the unattractive Campus buildings, began to overcast my life. I realised what was happening so I booked an appointment with Dr Grey, my new GP in Helensburgh, and although I got the earliest available appointment it still meant that I would miss my Maths lesson that morning. To be honest I wasn't that upset to be missing Maths, sure I would be behind and I would have to catch up on my studies but the real reason for me not being too upset was that I could not stand our teacher Jenny Tyler. Miss Tyler was one of the most cold hearted, unfeeling people that I have ever had the misfortune to meet. I, along with the rest of my class, witnessed her reducing a 35 year old woman to tears because she had made an error in her classwork. She was a mean spirited woman and the less I had to do with her the better. However, after I had missed a couple of her classes she decided that I was there to be made an example of and I took my place in class that morning feeling edgy and unaware of what was going to ensue.

Miss Tyler read out the registration and when she came to my name she halted abruptly.

"Suzy Johnston. Will you come out to the front please?"

I lifted my head from my hands which were folded on the white, Formica desk in front of me.

"Yeah, sure." I slouched my way to the front of the classroom.

She glared at me.

"Can you explain your absences over the past week?" she gesticulated angrily at the register.

"Yes. I'm really sorry but I had to see the doctor and..." She cut me off.

"See the doctor? See the doctor?! If you want to pass this course, which I doubt you will if you carry on like this, you are going to have to get your priorities straight and "seeing your doctor" shouldn't be one of them!"

"Hang on a minute, I really needed to see the doctor." I was struggling to keep my temper.

"Priorities Suzy, priorities. Your dedication to this course seems to be lacking. I'm in two minds whether to recommend that you should not be allowed to attend your teaching practice at nursery school next week. Believe me, if it was up to me you wouldn't be going! Now go and sit down!" The woman was nearly spitting at me. I turned and walked back to my seat noting the open mouths of my classmates.

"And where exactly do you think you are going?"

"Back to my seat." I answered confused.

"I think it would be better if you sat over at the other side of the classroom today."

I couldn't believe that she was so desperate to humiliate me by treating me like a seven year old and moving me away from my friends but I decided to just take it and not give her the satisfaction of an argument. Staring her straight in the eye I picked up my bag, walked over to an empty seat and sat down. Of course my health was my priority but to get into a discussion about that would have to have meant disclosing what my health problem was and, to be frank, Jenny Tyler was the last person I would want to have know about it.

My nursery placement went extremely well but by that point I was already beginning to question whether my future belonged in teaching. I enjoyed being with the kids and had fun helping to teach them about colours and shapes but I didn't enjoy having to constantly justify on paper what I was doing and make sure every "i" was dotted and "t" crossed. I was finding teaching too regimented and limiting and whilst I recognised the value of lesson plans I felt that they were at the expense of spontaneity and creativity (one of my tutors actually told me off for being too creative!). Unfortunately, like most people, when I was doing something that I didn't enjoy I became more and more unhappy and began to dread going to school. On top of everything else I was dog tired as I was up until two or three most mornings getting my lessons prepared or finishing off some assignment for class. I was depressed and struggling and it was just a question of where rather than when I would crack.

I was especially nervous that Tuesday morning as I knew that a Tutor from Jordanhill was coming in to observe me taking a class. I had been up until the early hours preparing and perfecting the lesson that I was going to teach but when I awoke on that morning I was exhausted and feeling really down. I sat in the car on the way to school silently counting the trees that flashed past noting miserably that each one brought me closer to school and closer to my Tutor visit. I wished, not for the first time that morning, that I was dead. As I struggled to keep things in perspective and pretend that everything was okay we pulled into the school car park and I saw Jenny Tyler getting out of her car. "Oh God, not her." I prayed "Not her." God wasn't listening and Jenny told us that she would observe first me then Gloria, the other student at the school. My class was a disaster, I'm the first to admit it. I gave out the worksheets that I had prepared and then retreated inside my head into my own little world away from such antagonists as school children, worksheets and Jenny Tyler. My body was present but the rest of me was long gone. Everything seemed to go into slow motion and I was having trouble connecting with reality. My thoughts felt jumbled and the classroom and everyone in it seemed very far away. Yes, I decided as I wandered aimlessly around the room, I like it like this. At the end of the lesson the sound of Jenny Tyler's biting tones brought me back to earth. She said she wanted to speak to me and would see me in the corridor. The purpose of Tutor visits, we had been told repeatedly, was not to criticise our work but to give us support and guidance. Someone had obviously forgotten to tell this to Jenny as she stood in the corridor, busy with passing pupils and teachers, telling me at the top of her voice about all my failings and how she doubted that I would ever be a decent teacher. She finished off her verbal assault by proclaiming that she could have pulled in anyone off the street and they would have done a better job than me. Fair enough, I thought, but where was the guidance, the support? Any idiot with glasses surely would have spotted that there was something far wrong with me that morning and asked what was going on. But for Jenny the fact that I had done a bad job was too good an opportunity to miss and she seemed to relish tearing me to pieces. It was the final nail in the coffin of my teaching career. I knew there and then that it was finished and I felt a huge

138

release inside me as months of repressed misery gushed out. I managed to hold the tears back until Jenny had left; I wasn't giving her the satisfaction.

I talked my decision over with my parents and they immediately supported my choice. They weren't blind and had seen how unhappy I had become over the past few months and were relieved that I had decided to leave the course. I also had a long chat with Dr Grey and whilst she was disappointed that I was giving it all up she realised the reasons for my decision. I went and saw Frank James, the course leader, the following day and made my intentions clear. He was a kind man and said he was sorry that I had decided to leave as he felt that I had a rosy future in teaching (he had observed one of my previous classes and given me a wonderful report.). He asked if there was anything about the course that I would like to comment on, some way that they could improve things. I thought about Jenny Tyler and bit my lip. Then I thought "Fuck it, I'm doing this for my classmates" and told Frank about my experiences of Jenny both in and out of the classroom. He was horrified and said he had had his suspicions but unfortunately there was nothing he could do. He paused. Unless, he said, someone was to write an official letter of complaint documenting her behaviour. As course leader he couldn't tell me to do this but if such a letter were to appear on his desk he would be forced to act on it. I nodded, shook his hand and bid him farewell.

As a matter of postscript I wrote that letter, Jenny received a verbal warning and transformed overnight into a much more pleasant and helpful tutor. My former classmates were extremely grateful!

CHAPTER 14

Things were not going well. Since leaving college my mood, rather than lifting, had hit an inexorable slide and I felt as though I was losing control. I was finding it nearly impossible to maintain any sort of conversation and as a result seemed to be pushing the people I cared about further and further away. I hated myself and tortuous minutes stretched into hours and hours into days. My only respite was sleep but that was fleeting and I would lie for hours during both day and night staring at the ceiling desperately looking for a way out. I wanted this to stop. I wanted to go and get a hug from my Mum and to be able to have a chat and a laugh but all that seemed a long, long way away and completely out of my reach at the present time. Crying would have been a relief and would at least have given my parents a clue as to how I was feeling but that too was something that had been robbed from me and I was left feeling violated and alone. I had even lost my long standing ability of being able to put on a protective outer "shell" to disguise how I was feeling, it simply took too much energy and the apathy that ran through my blood stream wouldn't allow it and laughed at me when I tried.

I had been seeing either Dr Grey or Dr Bradshaw the practice's newest doctor, basically whomever I could get an appointment with, and on that Wednesday morning I was due to see Dr Bradshaw at 10:30am. Dr Bradshaw, a petite young woman with long, dark hair neatly tied back, came out of her office into the calming pastel shades of the waiting room and called my name. I stood and followed her into her room. She asked me a few questions which I answered in a subdued voice and then said something which took me completely by surprise:

"How would you feel about spending a few days in hospital?"

I didn't know what to say. I was completely flummoxed. If someone had asked me whether I preferred strawberry or vanilla ice cream it would have taken me an age to answer never mind a question of this magnitude.

"I...uh...I don't know." I stuttered.

"A new psychiatric ward, the Christie Ward, has just opened in the Vale of Leven hospital and I really think it would do you some good to go there for a rest. What do you think?" she asked leaning forward in her chair.

"I really don't know...I just don't know."

"Take a few moments to think about it." She said and sat back in her chair.

I didn't know what to say. I didn't know what to say. I was totally confused and unsure of how to respond. I wished that someone else were here to make the decision for me. Psychiatric hospital? Fucking hell. But maybe this was what I needed, nothing else seemed to be working and I couldn't see myself getting well at home, maybe, like Dr Bradshaw said, it would be a good idea. I mentally crossed my fingers and took the plunge.

"Okay" I said breaking the silence. "I'll do it. I'll go."

"Good. Just hang on a minute until I make a few phone calls." she smiled and picked up the phone receiver on her desk.

I left the surgery feeling a little in shock and having been told that the Christie Ward was expecting me at 5:00pm. Now I had to break the news to my family. How would they take it? I was sure they had

142

never expected one of their children to end up in a psychiatric ward and I was already feeling the guilt of letting them down. My parents and brothers were kind, loving people but I was just about to drop a whole heap of stress on them and I was unsure of how they would react. "Please be okay" I prayed; I didn't think I had the energy to handle a family crisis at that point.

My Mum was stunned when I told her the news of my impending admission and immediately burst into floods of tears. It's not often that one sees your Mum crying and I felt awful for having been the cause of it. I didn't know what I could say to reassure her and I hated myself even more. My younger brother, Ollie, was much calmer and arranged for a friend to come and take me down to her house until my Mum had calmed down. Then he sat Mum down, made her a coffee and called one of her best friends, Shona, explained what had happened and said "Mum's having a twenty minute wobble but she'll call you in thirty minutes for a chat."

I was sitting drinking tea at Isobel's house when I received a call from Mum saying "I'm fine now and I'm ironing your pyjamas. If you're going into a psychiatric ward you're bloody well going to look smart! Don't worry we're all right behind you and we love you heaps."

The Christie Ward is situated at the side of the Vale of Leven Hospital where the nurses' quarters used to be. It is a custom built facility with 24 beds divided into either 4 bedded dorms or single rooms, both dorms and rooms having en suite facilities. There are also two staff offices, reception, two kitchens (one for occupational therapy work and one for staff), a "quiet" room, a dining room, a TV room (or the "smoke room" as it is known-patients are allowed to smoke there), several interview rooms, two bathrooms, a laundry, the main meeting room, where Multi Disciplinary Team meetings (or "reviews") take place once a week and, when weather permits, a small back garden with garden furniture where patients can get some fresh air. The Ward is set out in a rough "L" shape with the meeting point of the two branches being at the reception area that is overlooked by the staff room.

(I feel that it is important to note that my admissions to the Christie Ward are remembered with the assistance of those close to me as my memory of those times is extremely poor due to the obvious fact that I was so ill.)

I had the rather dubious honour of being one of the first patients admitted to the Ward as it had only been open for a few days and as a result it was less than half full when I arrived. I remember standing in reception with my parents feeling very nervous and vulnerable – the place didn't look like and certainly didn't smell like a hospital and I wasn't sure what to make of it. So I stood there in silence holding my little case waiting for whatever was going to happen next. A dark haired female nurse holding a clipboard appeared through an open door and smiled at us. She showed my parents and me through to one of the four bedded dorms and indicated which bed would be mine. Then, referring to her clipboard, she asked me a whole heap of questions which I answered as well as I could in the circumstances. She tried to reassure my unspoken worries and the visible fear in my face by telling me that this was not a place to be scared of and that if I had any concerns I could approach a nurse at any time day or night. She asked me if I had brought some things from home and I answered "Yes" and motioned towards my case. She picked it up and, laying it

144

on the bed, explained that she would have to look through my belongings firstly to take an inventory of the items in it and secondly to see if there were any "Sharpies" - things that might be considered dangerous and not allowed on the Ward. Bemused I nodded my agreement and before I knew it my leg razors and glass bottle of moisturiser were whipped away to be placed in a locked cupboard far away from my reach. I was feeling tremendously insecure and unsure of my surroundings and I clung to my parents for support hoping somehow that their confidence and easy manner would rub off on me. We were then shown around the Ward and I glanced anxiously at the other patients that we encountered sure, at that moment, that none of them would like me and that they would make it as difficult as possible for me to survive in that place. My parents left me with hugs and reassurance that they would be back to visit tomorrow. I didn't let them know how I was feeling as I didn't want to add to the already copious amount of stress that I had placed on them already so once they were gone I drew the curtain around the bed, sat on the bed and, staring at the floor, imagined that I was the only person in the World and that nothing could harm me. I stayed there in my own little world, mindless of the cramp in my bum, for four hours when a nurse popped her head around the curtain and said that the Doctor was ready to see me now. I nodded, stretched and followed the nurse out into the corridor and into one of the interview rooms. The nurse left and I talked a little to this strange Doctor whom I had never seen before in my life. I didn't know him, I certainly didn't trust him and I was supposed to tell him everything about me and how I was feeling? I didn't think so. So I admitted to feeling depressed and having some suicidal thoughts but that was about it. I wouldn't, couldn't tell him about the feelings of isolation and fear that were with me all the time, the continual preoccupation with ways of killing myself and the way that I hated myself so damn much.

I returned to my room, of which I was the only occupant, and decided to see for myself if this Ward was as suicide proof as it claimed to be. I checked the windows first; unbreakable and they only opened about 10cms. Hmm. Nothing to hang yourself from; the curtain rail had a look of deliberate flimsiness about it and the mirrors were also unbreakable, metal instead of glass. How did I feel? Relief. Like a huge weight had been lifted from my shoulders. Here was a place where I could live and not have to constantly think that, if I wanted, I could jump out of a window, or smash a mirror and slash my wrists or hang myself or any number of ways that I could kill myself. It was impossible in here and the suicide factor had mercifully been taken out of the equation.

I spent the next few days settling in and getting used to the hospital routine; when mealtimes were etc. but kept myself to myself on the whole. I started to talk a little at mealtimes to a patient named Anne who was in the Ward because of a failed suicide attempt – she had walked into the hills wearing only t-shirt and shorts in a still chilly April, chased a bottle of pills with some vodka and lain down to die. Luckily some hill climbers had literally tripped over her and called an ambulance. Anne was noticeable in the Ward because she wore scrubs, as she had no belongings with her, so I asked my Mum to bring in some toiletries with her so that Anne could have a few possessions of her own.

I had been in the Ward a couple of days and was sitting hunched up on my bed talking to my Mum when a nurse came into the room. I hadn't seen her before and she was noticeable for her unruly black hair. She was dressed in casual clothes, as all the nurses were, and asked if she could sit down. When I nodded she pulled up a chair and introduced herself "Hi, I'm Emma. I'm going to be your Named Nurse." I couldn't have cared if she had said she was going to be Superman, I wasn't interested in talking to her and I'm sure my negative body language conveyed this impression. However, never one to be deterred Emma sized up the situation and continued.

"I'm going to be responsible for your care whilst you're in the Christie Ward. When you feel more like it we can have a talk about how you're feeling and draw up a Care Plan for you. Whenever I'm on duty you can come and have a chat with me. I'll be there for you, okay? If you have any questions about the role of a Named Nurse this leaflet should answer them." She handed my Mum the leaflet. " Any questions now?"

Silence from me.

"Okay. Well I'll come back later on, I can see you're busy talking to your Mum. I'll see you later."

I didn't know it then but I was extremely lucky to have been appointed Emma as my Named Nurse. She was, and is, an exceptionally capable, intelligent and caring nurse with a wicked sense of humour and it took her only a short while to break down my stony defences and cajole me into talking. She would take me for walks and spend a lot of her time with me and says now that I would talk about anything other than how I was feeling. I relied on my tactic of deflecting what was being asked and turning around to ask the questioner about his or, in this case, her life. However I had underestimated Emma's intelligence and savvy and she was too smart

147

to be sucked in by my ploy. It must have been frustrating for her but she persevered and wouldn't give up on me. It is to her credit that I don't remember exactly when I started letting her into my lonely, miserable world – it just kind of crept up on me and before I knew it I was opening up the creaky doors of my inner self and sharing my thoughts with this new and valuable confidant. I soon discovered that Emma was impossible to shock and this gave me the confidence to broach subjects that had previously gone unspoken to anyone.

The Ward quickly began to fill up and there began to be a real sense of community amongst the patients; we all supported each other and tried to make life as easy for each other as well so when Neil, a gentle, kindly man had to go to court because he had stabbed two trespassing boys during a psychotic episode we wished him all the best and crossed our fingers for him. We were all ill and regardless of upbringing and background we all had a common bond and had a huge amount of empathy for each other. I tended to sit at the back of the smoke room on my own but the other patients were quick to include me in their conversations and encouraged me to join them. I didn't have to explain my reticence, nothing was expected of me, and I was happy just to sit amongst company without the added pressure of having to tell my life story. Of course, there was the odd patient who was hard to get along with, most notably Zandra – a very ill young woman who would constantly bug unwell patients for cigarettes; even when she had plenty of her own, and was not averse to rummaging through others' drawers.

I remember being ashamed of myself one day when the German doctor on the Ward had upset one of the patients and racist insults were being hurled around the smoke room. Normally, when I was well, I would have said something to stop the abuse but I was simply too ill to make a stand on my own and instead I slunk out of the room and retreated to my bed. Avoidance seemed the best policy but I still felt guilty and as though I was condoning that behaviour.

Once a week each patient had the opportunity to talk with their psychiatrist in their MDT or "review". These meetings took place in the large meeting room and were attended by any number of SHOs, Occupational Therapists, Nurses, Social Workers and CPNs that were involved in your case. The first time I walked into a review I had no idea what to expect and I was horrified to see so many people in the one room. Immediately my coping mechanism sprung into action and I clammed up, staring at the floor to avoid inquisitive eyes. I mumbled answers to my psychiatrist's, Dr Blake's, questions and was desperate to be out of there and back to the safety of my bed as quickly as possible. I haven't a clue what was said or decided although it became apparent then, and in consequent reviews, that I wasn't to be discharged for the foreseeable future. Even now that I am older and better aware of how these things work I still dread reviews. I find them intimidating and uncomfortable and any negative feelings that I might have about myself seem to magnify in that environment. It would appear to be a much better idea for the psychiatrist to see the patient on his or her own and then report back to the multitudes that wait in the next room thereby sparing the patient the terror of facing so many people. Even when I am feeling better and approaching discharge I find reviews difficult and feel that I don't represent myself well so you can appreciate what a colossal nightmare they are for me when I am ill.

Before I had been admitted to the Christie Ward I had been seeing a psychologist, Mrs Watt in order to help me deal with how I was coping with my illness. I had enjoyed meeting with Mrs Watt and looked forward to our appointments where we talked about life, death, philosophy and metaphysics as well as manic depression and the problems it caused me. We also, on occasion, talked briefly about issues in her life which pleased me as I found her openness interesting and I appreciated the trust that she was paying me. It was decided, then, that whilst I was in hospital and under supervision it would be a good opportunity for Mrs Watt to supervise a program to be run under her guidance by Emma that would strip me of all of my "faulty" defence strategies and replace them with "healthy" ones. As far as I am aware everything was going well until approximately halfway through the course Mrs Watt decided to go on holiday and withdrew her guidance from the program. This left me, and Emma, in the shit. Emma tried her best to help me as much as possible, even reading up on psychology books during her time off and if it hadn't been for her I don't know how I would have ended up. Mrs Watt had abandoned ship right at the point where I had no defences and this left me extremely vulnerable and I took several large steps backwards on the road to recovery. I remember that Dr Blake was furious with the course of events and ordered a meeting at which Emma, Mrs Watt, myself and Dr Blake were to attend to try and discover what had gone wrong. I was terrified. I was extremely worried that somehow this was all my fault and all the blame would be laid at my door plus I was concerned that Mrs Watt was plotting against me and hated me. I didn't sleep at all the night before the meeting. Fortunately Emma was on duty and talking with her managed to take

150

the edge off my fear. She reassured me that she would be there, nobody would be out to get me and that she personally would come and get me when the meeting started. I tried to cling onto her words of comfort but they fell through my hands like dry sand and I was left frightened and ill equipped to cope with any sort of confrontation.

I spent an age getting dressed the following morning staring at my clothes trying to decide which top or which pair of trousers would ensure that the meeting went well. I didn't want to go. I really didn't want to go. I wanted to stay in my bed with the duvet pulled over me and all the lights switched off and for everyone to leave me alone. Not for the first time I wished that I could somehow be beamed forward two hours and have the meeting behind me so that I could make some attempts at getting back to leading a normal life. The second hand on the clock on the wall clicked unsympathetically forward. I swallowed some tea for breakfast and bummed a cigarette off my friend Julie and then sat smoking and chewing my nails in the smoke room. The tension was almost unbearable and I wanted to scream and scream and scream. But I didn't. Instead I paced the corridors mumbling words of comfort to myself and by the time Emma came to get me I was sitting on my bed hugging my knees feeling like a condemned woman.

I like to write poetry and find that, especially when I'm depressed, it's a valuable outlet for my emotions and I can often put down on paper what I can't say in word. I had written a poem the day before and I had discussed with Carrie, another nurse, whether I should show it to Dr Blake at the meeting as I felt it represented quite well how I was feeling. She thought that that was a good idea so armed with my poetry book I followed Emma down the corridor to the main meeting room.

The meeting was brutal. It began with me showing my poem to Dr Blake and then he passed it to Mrs Watt who casually flicked through the entire book much to my anger. She then told me that she thought I was acting like a thirteen year old by the way that I presented the poem to Dr Blake. Immediately I could feel the self protection shutters coming down but was determined to retain my composure and answer her challenges to the best of my ability. More abuse followed. After that I have no recollection of what happened; I think I've blocked it out but I do know that after I left the room Dr Blake gave Mrs Watt a bollocking for the way that she spoke to me and was furious with how she had handled the entire situation. I couldn't really care I was just so relieved to have the meeting behind me and when Emma came to find me I was lying on my bed feeling relaxed for the first time in days.

"I bet you're glad that's over." She smiled "You okay?"

I sat up "That was horrible. Horrible." I made a face.

"Are you angry with me for not speaking up for you?" Emma looked serious.

"No"

"Are you sure? It's okay you know."

"Well, maybe, just a little bit. Why didn't you help me? I thought you were on my side."

"I am on your side, I just thought that you were doing fine on your own and that if I jumped in it might detract from what you were saying. So I left you to it and you did great."

"I didn't feel great just hugely intimidated. I could hardly squeeze the words out."

"Well don't worry it's over and believe me Dr Blake tore a strip off Mrs Watt that she won't forget for a long time. C'mon let's go and get a cup of tea, I think we deserve it."

Emma had been on duty all through the previous night from 7.15pm to 7.15am and she was still here at 11.30am just so that she could attend that meeting with me. Yet another thing to add to the long list of things I owe her.

I was still a secret smoker. I only smoked in the smoke room when the nurses weren't around and I was constantly worried that someone might casually mention to one of my parents that I smoked. Eventually I realised how stupid I was being and decided that it was time to own up and tell my Mum about my habit; after all I was 23, what could she say? She arrived that afternoon bright and breezy as ever bearing some freesias, my favourite flower, and after popping her head in the nurses office for a quick chat walked into my room. We embraced and talked for a short while. Then I suggested that we go down to the hospital's tea bar for a coffee. C'mon Suzy keep your nerve. After I checked that it was okay for me to leave the Ward we headed down stairs to the tea bar and ordered a couple of demon strength coffees and a cake each. We chatted about this and that until suddenly I could stand it no more and blurted out:

"Mum, I've got two things to tell you!"

She looked at me quizzically and paused for a second. "Okay, what is it?"

I took a deep breath. "I smoke. I'm a smoker. I smoke cigarettes."
I waited for her reaction.

"Well okay, fair enough, you're old enough to decide these things for yourself. Don't worry, I'm not cross and come to think of it I'm not that surprised either. What's the second thing?"

My breath exploded out of me "Can you get me twenty Marlboro Lights when you're next in visiting?!"

My Dad dropped the fags in that night when he came to visit. He's a smoker himself and tried hard but couldn't suppress the chuckle that escaped from his lips when he handed them over. Later that week I was home on a pass for the afternoon and smoked my first cigarette in front of my parents. It was dreadful - I was really nervous about it and smoked the thing so bloody fast that I nearly passed out! My Dad was now my partner in crime and we would spend many evenings smugly smoking fags with me making pathetic attempts at smoke rings.

I'm lucky to have such a great father. He's kind, thoughtful and most importantly brings me cheeseburgers from McDonald's with him when he comes to visit which is a welcome respite from hospital food! He is also in possession of a wicked sense of humour: one day I was due to fly out to Majorca for a Summer holiday and Dad was keeping me company at the head of a very long and impatient passport queue. He gave me a parting hug and whispered in my ear "Watch this." Then, at the top of his voice, yelled "Fine! Go on your own then!" and stormed off! Everyone in the queue stopped what they were doing and stared at my reddening face. Dad was killing himself laughing. Bastard! Actually, I have to admit that it was pretty funny even if it did rate about eleven on the embarrassment scale!

Dad found my illness very difficult to handle at first. Here was something that he couldn't fix or be cured by a hug or a kind word and I think he found my reclusiveness hurtful. When I was a kid I had a blue sweatshirt that had "Daddy's Wee Dear" emblazoned on it but Daddy's wee dear was long gone and in the grip of a depression it must have seemed like I was deliberately shutting him out – I would hardly speak to him and feel resentful of his cheerfulness. I love my Dad. I really do, but I think both of our hearts were bruised during that time and for that I'm sorry.

Gradually, however, like the good parent he is he began to understand my illness. He was, and is, determined not to lose me even when I was feeling lost and alone. I know now that he is always there for me and is someone |I can rely on and turn to regardless of the circumstances. He is a strong man and will always be there to prop me up when things are bad.

One of my biggest, nagging fears is that all of the men on my Dad's side of the family have died at a relatively young age from heart attacks and whilst my Dad, fortunately, remains healthy I want him to know how much I value my time with him and how fortunate I am to have such a kind, loving man as a father.

During my first stay in the Christie Ward I was embarrassed at my naivety of the drug culture that is so prevalent in our society. It was brought home to me extremely abruptly the destructive effects that illegal drug use can have on the mind and a significant percentage of patients were admitted for precisely that reason. When I look at the zombied face of Jeremy or listen to the psychotic ramblings of Martha I wonder whether that "hit" was really worth it and whether they had ever considered the ramifications of their actions at the time. It occurred to me sometime after my discharge that whilst we are, on the whole, aware of the negative physical effects the drug use can have on the body little is made of the equally debilitating psychological or psychiatric problems that can arise. True, a psychological illness may not actually kill you but it may well persuade you that jumping off a bridge is a good idea and a life spent in a psychiatric hospital when it might otherwise have been productive is surely equally tragic. My heart went out to Kirsten during the very visible agonies of her drug withdrawal, a withdrawal that made my previous experience look like a walk in the park, and it was me she decided to turn to when she had smuggled a knife out of the dining room. She was contemplating slashing her wrists to escape the mental anguish that hounded her like an angry dog twenty four hours a day seven days a week. We talked and eventually she decided to turn the knife in to one of the nurses and a crisis was averted. I was left shaking and terrified that if I had somehow said the wrong thing to her it all might have turned out horribly differently. I was too fragile to handle the responsibility and too weak to make major decisions for myself, never mind someone else.

Whilst the Ward was not the happiest place to be the nurses did their best to lighten the atmosphere and it was not without its moments of humour which shone like jewels in the sun in a rather bleak landscape. I was wandering down one of the corridors one morning lost in thought when I bumped into Carrie, one of the nurses.

"Are you feeling depressed today, Suzy?" she asked looking concerned.

"Yeah." I mumbled

"I'm not surprised. I'd be depressed if I had a spot like that on my nose!" she chuckled and nudged me with her arm.

That comment brought a smile to my face that had been absent for quite some time and helped me to realise that, in a small way, there was hope and a little light cracked through at the end of my tunnel.

Another humorous incident occurred when, one evening, I was sitting in the smoke room having a cigarette and talking to Kirsten. It was around 10:30pm and the "drug trolley" from which we received our night time medication was due. Emma and Valerie were amongst the nurses on duty that night and it was the two of them that appeared outside the smoke room with the trolley. Getting night time meds is a personal thing; some people like to queue whilst others prefer to wait until their name is called. I was a "queue-er" and patiently stood in line until it was my turn. Valerie handed me a small, plastic cup with my pills inside and another one filled with water. I gave my pills a cursory look and was about to take them when I suddenly stopped. I took a closer look at my pills and, yes, there amongst the usual antipsychotic and mood stabilisers was a large purple pill that I had never seen before.

"What's this?" I asked poking the purple pill.

"Come on Suzy, just take your meds," said Emma looking serious.

"No way, not until you tell me what this pill's for. It's huge!"

"Suzy, take your pills! There's people waiting," chipped in Valerie.

"Tell me what it's for."

Emma folded her arms. "If you don't take your pills we'll have to write you up as refusing to take them and you don't want that do you?"

"Just tell me what it is."

Emma leaned over and whispered conspiratorially in my ear

"It's a jellybean. Blackcurrant I believe." And started chuckling

"You swines. The pair of you!" I laughed and promptly ate the chewy and tasty sweet.

By this point everyone in the drug queue was laughing and we all felt like regular people enjoying a good joke than psychiatric patients and nurses. For a few moments we forgot our problems and just laughed; it was a liberating experience and a brief respite from our inner torments.

CHAPTER 15

I was discharged after being in the hospital for three months. Three tough, long months in which I had learned the valuable lesson of being able to open up and talk to people about my fears and concerns. Although things weren't perfect (when are they ever?) I felt nervous and a little afraid but better able to cope with what life outside the hospital had to offer. The conditions of my discharge were that I see Leanne Hutton, a CPN, regularly and, obviously, take my medication. So I said my goodbyes, wished everyone all the best and deposited the largest box of chocolates that I could find in the nurses' office. I found Emma and tried my best to be eloquent and somehow thank her for all that she had done for me but I fumbled the words and ended up just giving her a big hug. Oh well. I walked out of the door with cries of "We hope we never see you here again!" ringing in my ears and carried my case down to the car where Mum was waiting.

The next few days were difficult. I felt incredibly exposed and vulnerable now that the protective shield of the Ward had disappeared. I was on my own and still recovering from the institutionalisation that had crept up on me during my admission. I was too used to the hospital routine and was missing the opportunities that I had to talk to a nurse or see a doctor whenever I needed to. I panicked and phoned the Ward only to be reassured that Leanne would be out to see me in the next couple of days. I stuck close to my Mum nervous of what people would think of me now that I had been in a psychiatric ward although my friend from my Jordanhill days, Liz, reckoned that as I had been discharged from a psychiatric ward I was officially declared sane and it was everyone else that I should be worried about!

Leanne came to visit after a few days and I liked her immediately. She was bright, wise, funny and had a sort of down to earth quality about her. I found her easy to talk to and after our first chat she suggested that I go with her to a Manic Depression Fellowship meeting that was taking place that Tuesday in Glasgow. She picked me up in her car and we headed for Glasgow arriving at our destination, The Charlie Reid Centre just shy of 7:30pm. As we were getting out of the car Leanne told me that as it was my first visit all I would have to do would be introduce myself and if I didn't fancy speaking after that that was okay. I agreed that that was fine with me too and we climbed the steps to the front door. As we entered the front door we were met by a good looking man in his early thirties. He introduced himself as Dan and explained to me that he would be facilitating the meeting. He took us through to the meeting room and invited us to sit down. I glanced round the room trying not to stare at the other people that were present. There were both male and female, young and old and everyone was chatting loudly sharing experiences that had happened over the past couple of weeks since the last meeting. Then Dan called for quiet and everyone took a seat and a hush descended over the room. One by one everyone introduced themselves saying their name and explaining a little about their current circumstances. Suddenly I realised that it was my turn and with a supportive look from Leanne said "Hi, my name's Suzy. I have manic depression and I have just been discharged from hospital."

"How long were you in for?" asked a man with a grizzled beard and glasses.

"Three months." I replied

"Which hospital were you in? Gartnaval?"

"No, the Vale of Leven, the Christie Ward. It's new." I offered by way of explanation.

The meeting moved on and it became apparent that the main topic of conversation that evening was going to be the quality of hospital care and I was interested to hear other people's experiences to compare them to my own. However after listening to those people speak for about twenty minutes I was growing more and more horrified and angry. All of the experiences offered were extremely negative and no one had even the vaguest good word to say about life in a psychiatric ward. I had to say something so, sidestepping my shyness, I opened my mouth and said:

"Look, I can appreciate that most of you seem to have had horrendous times in hospital but I've just been discharged from a new facility and I feel that it was a positive experience that has made me a stronger person. The Ward was well equipped and the staff were enthusiastic, caring and supportive. I don't know where I would be without their help and I find it reassuring that if I ever become that ill again, and I pray I won't, that the Christie Ward is there to help me recover. There are good hospitals and nurses out there and I can't sit here and let you say otherwise."

Amongst the mutterings of "There's always a lucky one" some people were interested and keen to hear about a ward that opposed their views so I explained about my time in the Christie Ward and about how it helped me. Maybe it offered them some hope, I don't know, but it certainly reinforced in me how bloody lucky I had been not to end up in one of their nightmares.

161

After the meeting I spent a few minutes talking with Dan before heading home in the car with Leanne. As we escaped the ever hectic city she asked me what I had thought and I replied that, on the whole, I had enjoyed the meeting and that it was encouraging to meet so many people with manic depression that were getting on with their lives. However, I was saddened to hear of so many terrible experiences at the hands of the health service and I was acutely aware of my good fortune. She smiled and nodded. I then added that I would like to go back to the next meeting and see how things progressed from there. Leanne thought that that was a good idea although she explained that as she wouldn't be able to make the next meeting would I be okay going on my own? I thought for a moment before answering "Yeah, I think so." She smiled again.

If I had thought that things between Pete and me would have improved during my enforced three month absence from the Alkahounds I was to be sadly mistaken. If anything things were worse and this was brought violently home to me when, during an argument, he grabbed me by the throat and pinned me against a wall. Now Pete's a big guy and as there was no one else in the room to ask for help I reacted instinctively and made as though to punch him in the face. At the last second I opened my hand and ended up slapping him. Hard. He let me go and I spent the rest of the day feeling guilty for having hit him. Of course, in retrospect I did exactly the right thing but at the time I felt terrible, as though I was the one in the wrong.

Another event occurred which wasn't violent but far more worrying. We had spent the day recording a new demo in the studio. The producer who was helping us record it was Simon, an affable man

162

with long hair in his late twenties. I was having a bit of a laugh with Simon sharing some jokes and banter and I noticed in a corner of my mind that Pete was getting quieter and quieter. Soon it was time to go home and I had arranged to give both Pete and Simon a lift back to their houses. However, a sullen Pete insisted that he wanted to get the bus and my attempts to persuade him that he was being daft fell on deaf ears and he stubbornly insisted that he was going to take the bus home. Fine by me I thought walk if you want. So I gave Simon a lift to his place and headed back to Helensburgh thinking nothing of it. It wasn't until much later that I discovered that the reason Pete didn't want a lift was that he was hoping that Simon would attack, or even rape me, when I was alone with him in the car. He felt he was justified in feeling this way because as far as he was concerned, I had been acting "inappropriately" whilst we were recording by joking around with Simon. Furiously I told him that I acted no different with Simon than I did with anyone else and what the Hell did he think he was playing at? Angrily he said that "Glasgow girls don't act like that." I retorted that there was nothing wrong with my behaviour – I'm me and I act like me take it or leave it. It wasn't just the fact that he hoped that I was going to get attacked but the cold calculation behind it that sent an icy trickle of fear down my spine. I should have walked away there and then. That would have been the sensible thing to do. But I didn't. I was sure that I could handle Pete and I was totally absorbed by the ever improving music that we were coming up with and it would have broken my heart to leave. Or maybe I just wasn't very sensible.

I decided that I needed to fill my days more with something that was stress free and fun an after talking it over with Leanne and looking around I began to volunteer at Knowetop Community Farm in Dumbarton, a nearby town. It was great and I enjoyed the fresh air; my jobs included, amongst other things, mucking out the cows and feeding the animals. The farm was small and easily managed by the three full time members of staff and volunteers like myself who spent a few hours a week lending a hand. An added bonus was that the farm was managed by Rachel who had taught me horse riding when I was a kid and had occasionally baby sat for me and my brothers. Rachel was great, a kind sensible person with a great sense of humour which filtered through the farm and made it a fun place to be, so much so that I began turning up at the farm on my days off. As Summer faded and Autumn and then Winter strode in to take its place the farm became a very cold place to work and an icy wind continually whipped around the stables and pens. I would arrive home red faced and with blue fingers eagerly anticipating the hot mug of tea that was waiting for me.

That Winter I began playing gigs with the band again and although things between my self and Pete were less than harmonious it didn't show on stage and, to all the punters that came to watch, onstage we were the best of friends. I have often been asked how, with all the problems with stress that I have, I can bring myself to stand, sing and play guitar in front of a smoky club filled with both friends and strangers? The answer is fairly basic; true, I get really nervous but when I am on stage if I'm having difficulties I just stare at the floor and pretend I'm in the studio rehearsing and that helps to calm me down. The biggest problem I have, though, is with my legs – they won't stop shaking – I must look like Elvis up there!

I had been a regular attendee at Manic Depression Fellowship (MDF) meetings since the summer and I was beginning to build some good friendships. Part of the attraction of the meetings was, I have to confess, Dan, and at the Christmas party I drank a few bottles of beer, summoned up all my courage, plonked myself down beside him and made a vague attempt at chatting him up. Fortunately he was receptive and we talked all evening. I found him highly entertaining and easy to talk to – basically he was just a lovely person and everything that I was looking for so I was delighted when he said that he would call me during the week.

I must have spent hours sitting in the bloody kitchen that week willing the phone to ring. Thankfully he did call and asked me if I would like to meet him for a drink in Glasgow that Saturday. It took me all of three seconds to reply that that would be lovely and I would see him then. At my suggestion we met in the rather dodgy "Nice and Sleazy's" (never has a club been so aptly named) mainly because I knew the club as I had played some gigs in it but we hastily moved on to the far more respectable CCA (Centre for Contemporary Art) which boasted a beautifully designed bar with trendy chairs and tables. We talked and laughed, both eager to find the other's jokes funny and when we felt more at ease broached a more serious subject that had been concerning both of us. We discussed whether it would be ethical for the two of us to "go out" and rationalised that as Dan, who worked as a psychologist, was not seeing me as a patient and that as both of our involvement with MDF was voluntary there should be no problem and happily the problem was resolved. After that we sat and talked for hours and when we finally parted I was giddy with infatuation and sang loudly in the car all the way home still slightly disbelieving of my luck.

I decided that I should tell Pete about Dan as he was bound to see him at a gig and I didn't want him finding out from anyone else. I thought that that would be pretty unfair so during a break in rehearsal when Paul and Rob had gone downstairs to buy some drinks from the café I told Pete as gently as I could that I was seeing Dan. He sat on the dirty, grey carpet in silence for a few moments and when I asked him if he had anything to say he replied "Yes. You're fired."

I was stunned. "Pardon?"

"You're fired. You can collect your things and go. Don't come back." He was staring at the wall in front of him refusing to look me in the eye.

"Hang on a minute, you can't just fire me because I'm going out with some guy. That's totally unfair!" Rob came bounding up the stairs.

"Coke for you Suzy, and Irn Bru for you Pete." He looked at Pete's stony face. "Everything okay?"

I smiled wanly "I've just been fired."

"Ha ha yeah right. Funny joke."

"I'm not kidding Rob, Pete's just fired me because I told him that I've started going out with this guy, Dan, and he can't handle it."

"Is this true Pete?" asked Rob

"Why not ask her, she seems to want to do all the talking." He answered brusquely.

"I'm going to get Paul," said Rob and disappeared downstairs. The two of us sat in silence and I gritted my teeth to hold back the fury that was building up inside me. How dare Pete dictate whether I could go out with someone or not! How dare he! He knew that I

166

wasn't interested in him, I had made that clear and now here he was telling me in a few short words that if Dan was to be my boyfriend I was out of the band, a band that I had poured my heart and soul into for three years. What a bastard! Surely if he cared for me or even loved me as much as he said he did he would want to put my happiness first and not mess with my head like he was doing now? Paul and Rob returned and I filled Paul in on what had happened as Pete was refusing to speak. Paul was horrified. I couldn't bear it any longer and as there was no way I was going to let myself cry in front of Pete I said "Fuck this. I'm going for a walk. You guys can sort this out." I stood up, grabbed my cigarettes and coat and headed out of the front door.

To this day I don't know what was said between the three of them but I can imagine that a few short words were exchanged. All I know for sure is that as I was making my way back to the studio after a twenty minute walk, time enough for my tears to dry and my eyes return to normal, Pete was waiting at the front door for me contrite and apologetic. He said he was sorry and that of course he wanted me to stay in the band. I fell for every word and suggested that he get some help, maybe counselling, as he obviously had some issues that needed resolving. He laughed and said "People like me, people from council estates don't go for help we just get on with it ourselves."

I told him that that was the biggest pile of bollocks that I had ever heard. I had met many people from similar backgrounds to his in the Christie Ward and they at least had the guts to face their problems head on and acknowledge that they needed help. He wouldn't listen and we returned inside with the issue unresolved.

Sometimes good things come out of the most unexpected situations and because of this confrontation with Pete I opened up to Paul about some of the incidents that had happened between us in the past. Paul was furious with me, and rightly so, that I hadn't mentioned them sooner. However, he made it clear that I could rely on him as a friend in the band and he would do his best to make sure that Pete and I were never left on our own again.

Unbeknownst to me Dan had spoken to my Mum and said that if necessary he would walk away if it came down to me making a decision between him and the band. He didn't want to cause me any problems and, unlike Pete, my happiness was his main concern.

Dan and I got on famously and he would come down to Helensburgh to spend most weekends with me. We never seemed to run out of things to talk about and we would speak to each other nightly on the phone and when Valentine's Day came around he took me to St Andrews for an extremely thoughtful and romantic weekend. Everything was going so well that I should have realised that there was something brewing around the corner that would upset everything. And it was all my fault. Shortly after we returned from St Andrews the destructive fog of depression began edging its way back into my life and as a consequence I began to be confused about what I wanted. I started to shut down emotionally and, as a form of self protection, began closing off relationships as I was becoming increasingly unable to cope with other people. I was frightened and thrashing around in a panic and in a moment of pure illogical reasoning decided that if I broke up with Dan this suffocating darkness would recede. So coldly and out of the blue I dumped him with no explanations or excuses. He was shaken but calm and quietly told me that I wouldn't get rid of him that easily and that he would always be there for me. I just wanted him to leave so that there would be one less person for me to deal with. I didn't feel relief I just felt nothing, an aching, desperate nothing that was beginning to consume me. Clinical depression can be a very self absorbing condition and everything external becomes difficult to cope with and, as a consequence, best to avoid. I was trying to find the words to explain how I was feeling but I felt hugely inept and ineloquent. My friend Hazel, who also suffers from manic depression, came over one evening to take me back to her house for a chat and a coffee. We talked for a while and I tried my best to explain the growing void in my head and the terrible thoughts that were lurking there. I confessed to her that I had been self harming again and, feeling absolutely no emotion, told her of my suicidal plans and ideas. She immediately called the hospital and then my parents explaining that she would take me over to the Christie Ward to be assessed as she felt that I was in an unsafe state of mind.

CHAPTER 16

I arrived at the familiar surroundings of the Christie Ward feeling numb and slightly disconnected from everything. I didn't know if I wanted to be here. I just didn't know and when a nurse came through to take me to see the on call doctor it felt as though she was talking to someone else and the real me was sitting quietly somewhere else observing the scenario. My parents arrived looking worried and slightly relieved at the same time. They knew now, better than I did, that I was in a place where I was safe and would recover and whilst they weren't exactly happy about it they were reassured. Mum had brought a case with her full of some of my things and I went through the expected admissions routine of having the case's contents checked for dangerous objects. I must confess that I felt a little violated and angry when I saw my razors being removed from my reach as I had been self harming frequently recently using it and the pain involved to help me reconnect with my fading emotions.

I was lucky to be given a single room and I valued the privacy that it gave me and the fact that it removed the necessity of having to speak to any room mates. I spent most of my time alone in my room, mainly to avoid other people, and after a week had past the psychiatrist told me that he would like me to smoke more! The reason for this seemingly ludicrous piece of advice was that the only place to smoke was the smoke room and as it was always busy with patients I would be forced to socialise a bit. I had been a little nervous about seeing Emma again as I felt a bit ashamed at being in the Ward again but she kindly reassured me that contrary to what I thought I hadn't let her down and explained that I was in the best place to get better. My

Named Nurse for that admission was Abigail, a tall, slim pretty nurse who was extremely capable and excellent at her job and as I knew her from my previous visit I felt confident in her abilities and was happy to have her as my Named Nurse.

I had started hallucinating again and was becoming increasingly frightened by the things that I saw. One night I looked at my watch and I would swear to this day that it said ten o'clock; in actual fact it was three o'clock in the morning. I decided that I was going to use the pay phone to give my Mum a call and was amazed to find that the floor had turned into water. After taking a few tentative steps I discovered that I could walk on it and phoned Mum to tell her of this incredible turn of events! Mum wisely kept me on the phone until a nurse came by to escort me back to my room reassuring me that the "water" was just blue lino and that as it was 3:00am I had better go back to bed and get some sleep. It wasn't so much that the things that I saw were scary it was just that they had no place being there. I think what bothered me most about it, though, was that I had no control over it and regardless of what I did the hallucinations could appear at any time. Sometimes when I was in my room on my own I would sit with my eyes tight shut scared of what I would see if I opened them. So when I saw a large grouse walking out of the wall I called Abigail and, panicking, explained what was going on. She reassured me that there was no grouse in the room and suggested that I bring up the topic of my hallucinations at the next review – a change in medication might help.

One afternoon I was sitting on my bed feeling extremely miserable and felt the familiar urge to self harm. I raked through my possessions finally pouncing on my hairbrush as a suitable weapon.

172

The hairbrush had thick, stiff, fake bristles and I found that if I rubbed it hard against the back of my hand it would cut through my skin with comparable ease. I was feeling so dead inside that the pain caused was almost pleasant in contrast and when I saw the blood I smiled; here was proof that I existed and was still alive. I was aware of myself breathing. I rubbed harder absorbed by the pain, blood and torn flesh only stopping when I realised that I had no way to hide the wound from the prying eyes of the nursing staff. Stupid, stupid, stupid, I chastised myself and walked to the toilet to get some paper towels to try and tidy up the mess. Abigail popped her head round the door and caught my simultaneously guilty yet defiant stare. Removing my hairbrush she took me through to the treatment room and cleaned and dressed my hand talking to me gently about my motivation for hurting myself. She pointed out that there were healthier ways of helping myself when I was feeling down. I replied that cutting myself was such an intense act that it was almost addictive and I felt that, at that time, I relied on it to get me through the worst times. I didn't know what else to do. Nothing else seemed to work. She countered that self harming is ultimately destructive and causes more problems than it might seem to cure. It was not a solution and my attitude to it had to be addressed. She took me back to my room and checked that there was nothing else there that I could use to hurt myself. There wasn't and I felt resentful and petulant, angry that my secret had been discovered and removed from me.

At the review that week Dr Blake decided to change my medication by switching the antipsychotic that I was on to another variety. I remember being pleased at this as I had heard good things about the drug and hoped that it would help me with the hallucinations and bad thoughts that I was having.

Dan had been coming to visit me almost every day - so much so that one of the longer term patients, Jeff, opened a book on how long it would take us to get back together! Dan and I were getting along really well and it was good having him around. He would write hilarious letters to me that helped to brighten my day and I began to question whether I had done the right thing by breaking up with him. I felt I could talk to him about anything and, once I had had a few sessions with Abigail, he was the person that I asked to dispose of my secret collection of razors that I had stashed at home.

As I entered my third week in the Ward I was feeling a lot better but began to have this slightly uncomfortable edgy feeling that was with me all the time and worse with each passing day. I put it down to the fact that I felt cooped up in the Ward and wanted to be at home so I didn't mention it either at my review or to the nurses. I figured that once I was discharged it would go and everything would be okay.

I was delighted to be discharged at the beginning of my fourth week in the Ward and Mum and Dan came to pick me up and take me home. It was great to be back home but I still couldn't shift the edgy feeling that I seemed to be carrying around with me. In fact it was getting worse and worse to the extent that I couldn't sleep and didn't want to leave the house. I would spend my days sitting in the kitchen smoking, drinking coffee and shaking from head to toe. It was mental torture and I can only describe it as being in a room with a thousand people screaming at me twenty four hours a day. Then I started to have breathing problems so Mum took me over to Casualty where the on duty doctor decided that the antipsychotic was causing the muscles in my diaphragm to spasm and making it hard for me to breathe. It was terrifying. I was also hallucinating with a much greater regularity, so much so that I moved into the spare room at home where the plain, white walls offered less of a threat. I was totally freaked out and didn't eat anything for three weeks. When I managed to grab a couple of hours of sleep I would wake up unable to catch my breath and then panic, which would exacerbate the whole situation. I was frantic and was too distressed to maintain any kind of conversation with people. Dan would come down to visit and would hold my shaking hand and sit with me in silence. My Mum booked me an appointment to see Dr Gray and I remember sitting in the car until the very minute of my appointment because there was no way that I could bear to be in the waiting room with all those other people. Dr Gray saw me for a few minutes before asking why I was shaking so much. I explained that it was the medication and told her how the past few weeks had been. She picked up the phone and demanded that Dr Blake see me immediately. I saw him that afternoon and was told that I would have to wait until there was a bed free in the Christie Ward before I could be admitted. So I spent three excruciating days, taking medication to knock me out and help me get rid of the hallucinations, at home waiting, waiting, waiting with Leanne doing her utmost to secure me a bed and keep me sane.

Finally a bed became available and I was admitted. Blood tests showed that I was malnourished and in poor physical shape (I had lost two stone) so, after seeing a dietician, I was put on a regime of utterly revolting build up drinks. If I had thought that I could leave my hallucinations at home I was mistaken and they continued to persecute me in the Ward so much that I asked if I could move out of my single room at the far end of the Ward and into a four bedded dorm so that I could have some company as I was feeling lonely and isolated.

To my intense relief Dr Blake took me off the antipsychotic that had been causing me such terrible problems and put me on another one that was reportedly much less likely to cause any difficulties. When the drug trolley came round that evening I swallowed the pills eagerly crossing my fingers that finally they had found a drug that would work for me. Surely things couldn't get any worse?

Once again Abigail was my Named Nurse and when I was feeling a little stronger she thought it would be a good idea for me to fill in a mood sheet so we could see how my mood was at different times of the day and gradually build up a log of how I was progressing. The mood charts were simple; they were graded on a scale from zero to ten where zero was feeling completely depressed and ten was feeling great. I agreed to fill them in and conscientiously wrote in the appropriate number every morning, afternoon and evening.

Gradually I began to socialise more in the Ward and started spending most of my time in the smoke room chatting with the other patients. My doctor on the Ward during that admission was Dr York, one of Dr Blake's SHOs and I found her approachable and easy to talk to. Whilst I wasn't exactly happy I felt that I was improving and my mood charts reflected this. So I was completely unprepared for the giant wrecking ball that was about to smash through my mind.

When I woke at 5:00am that morning I was badly frightened and my instincts told me to trust no one especially the Ward staff who were plotting against me. The delusions that I was suffering from; that I was evil, about to be thrown out of my home and a fraud, seemed as

176

real as the bed that I was sitting on. I rationalised that my only chance was to get myself discharged from the hospital. But how? The nurses weren't stupid and had probably realised how evil I was already. It was hopeless. Then I spotted the mood charts lying on top of my locker and a plan began to form in my confused mind: I would doctor the charts to make it look as though I was doing really well, not too well, I didn't want anyone to get suspicious, but well enough so that it would speed up my discharge. I got out my pen and started scoring out the threes and fours and replaced them with eights and nines, even the occasional ten. Then I got back into bed and pulled the duvet over my head and quietly sobbed my heart out. Whilst I was suffering these delusions life was Hell. Imagine that you are watching television and the pictures and sound are your thoughts and emotions. When the TV is working everything is nice and clear but imagine that a little interference appears on the screen; it is still possible to make out the picture but it takes a little effort. This is what it is like when the delusions start. Eventually it becomes impossible to make out anything as the interference takes over and the delusions are all you can think about all day, all the time. It took a tremendous effort to act normally in front of people and not scream out "I know you can see the evilness inside me! I know it!" I had to pre-plan everything that I said or did, spontaneity was out of the question. I had to remind myself to laugh when someone said something funny and not recoil when someone gave me a hug. It took a huge amount of self control and having to act naturally around the nurses whilst I was in the hospital was exhausting. I knew that they were planning to harm me. I KNEW it and I was desperate to get away. Finally, after three weeks in the Ward I was discharged after smiling my way through a review and reassuring everyone that I was fine. Whilst I hoped that life would get easier when I got home the reality was that things were going to get a whole lot worse.

I was living in a constant state of fear and terror. I watched the football World Cup final but took in nothing of the match as my inner self was consumed with worry that my parents were on the verge of throwing me out of the house leaving me penniless and destitute. For hours, weeks, months I agonised whether I should tell someone what I was thinking but as I was convinced that all of it was true there seemed no point. Seeing Dan was horrendous as I was sure that he believed that I was evil but was hiding it from me. I was frightened of him. Leanne came to visit weekly and somehow I held it together and told her that I was doing fine, fine, fine. The only thing that I admitted to was feeling really anxious as I couldn't hide my agitation from those around me. I saw my doctor and was put on some tranquillisers to try and calm me down. I would take one of the pills feel a little better for twenty minutes and then count the minutes until I could take another one. It was agonising and I was in a terrible, frantic state. I was desperate for a way out and I couldn't find one. I was wearing myself out and fast reaching the end of my tether. Finally, after waking up one morning to the realisation that here was another day to struggle through I decided that the solution that had been coming more and more to the fore was the only way out; I was going to have to kill myself. It was almost a relief to make that decision, to finally know that the screaming, condemning noise in my head was going to be quieted. I decided that I was going to take an overdose – there was plenty of medication in the house and I knew that most of it was potentially lethal when taken in large doses. But before I did that that little bit of me that was clinging onto life decided to confront my Mum and tell her that I knew of her plans and thoughts. I hung around her all morning trying to build up my courage to speak to her about what was going on in my head. Finally, in her bedroom she said

"Come on, out with it. Something's bothering you. In fact something's been bothering you for a while now so what's up?"

"Uuuh." I stuttered.

"What's the matter Suzy, it can't be that bad."

It all came out in a rush. "I know that you think that I'm a terribly evil person and that you and Dad are planning to kick me out of the house."

She looked stunned and big, fat tears started pouring down my cheeks.

"What? I mean , what? That's not the case at all! Oh my god is that what you think? Oh Suzy come here." She held out here arms.

"No wait." I gulped "That's not all. I'm a fraud Mum. A fake. There's nothing wrong with me, I'm not ill. It's all lies." I sat on the bed and covered my face with my shaking hands. She sat down beside me and put her arms around me.

"No, Suzy, you're ill. In fact I think you're more ill than any of us have realised. Now listen to me. Listen. You're not evil, Dad and I are not plotting to throw you out of the house and you're not a fake. Okay? You're not. Now I'm going to phone the Ward because I think you need to speak to a nurse."

If only delusions could be cured like that. A quick easy fix. But just because my Mum had said those kind words didn't mean that my warped thinking was suddenly cured. In fact all that happened was

179

that I now believed that she didn't see the whole truth and I was still an evil fraud. The things the mind can do to itself. I was running round in circles getting beaten back by walls of negative thought no matter which way I turned.

I cried down the phone to Jake, one of the Christie Ward nurses, and he basically reinforced what my Mum had said adding that he thought it would be a good idea if I saw Leanne as soon as possible. But by the time Leanne came to visit my self defence denial walls had sprung back up in their place and I told her that I felt fine now and that there was no problem. But Leanne was no fool and didn't fall for my "hey, I'm okay" front for a second. She questioned me closely and my flimsy put-on image cracked and, crying, I admitted what was going on in my head. I fully expected her to express her disgust for me and confirm that I was an evil person but she didn't. Instead she picked up the phone and called the Christie Ward to see if any beds were available. Fortunately there was and we were told that if we were quick I might be able to bag one. Mum hurriedly packed me a small case of overnight things, put me in the car and drove like a demon over to the Christie Ward.

I was so ill that the admission was a blur and all I remember was being told that as I was being admitted on a Tuesday I wouldn't see Dr Blake until the next review, the following Monday. I was horrified by this news as I knew it meant that my medication would not be altered for almost a week and, as I had begun to suspect in fleeting rational moments that my delusions were as a result of the antipsychotic that I was taking, this meant that I would have to endure another six whole days until anything could be done. I wasn't sure that I could manage it. One result of being back in hospital was that I was again in the close proximity of the nurses and as I still believed that they were plotting against me I became very frightened. Paradoxically, it was the nurses that I had been closest to, like Emma, Carrie and Valerie, that I had the biggest problem with to such an extent that my Mum asked, on my behalf, if Emma could stay away from me as I was terrified of her and just being in her presence brought me out in a cold sweat. I felt utterly despondent and wretched and frustrated that the suicide proof Ward offered me no easy escape. I couldn't bear being in my head a second longer but there was no way out so at aged twenty five I clung onto my Mum's hand and begged her to stay with me. Eventually, of course, she had to leave and prised herself from my grasp reassuring me that she would be back to see me tomorrow. She told me not to worry and that now that I was in the hospital I would start to get better. It would all be okay. But she didn't see the dangers that I did. Only I knew that the nurses and other patients could see the evil that festered inside me. Only I knew that there was absolutely nothing wrong with me and all of these doctors and nurses were mistaken. And only I knew how utterly terrified I was.

My first night in the hospital was difficult primarily because of my anxieties but also because my roommate, Sheila, was in the midst of a psychotic episode and continually yelled at me to press the "call" button in our room to summon the night staff. I can't recall who was my Named Nurse during that admission but I would meet with one nurse or another (except Emma) for a chat once a day. I told them that I didn't want to take my antipsychotic anymore as I was growing more and more certain that it was at the root of my problems. Talking with the nurses wasn't easy; my stomach would tie itself in knots and

I would try and keep the meetings as brief as possible. The nurses would explain over and over again that I needed to take my medication which, if necessary, would be reviewed at Monday's MDT. "You don't understand!" I wanted to scream "It's killing me! I can't stand this anymore!"

I asked the nurses to place a ban on any incoming calls for me and also to forbid any visitors except my Mum. This ban included my Dad, my brothers and Dan. I just couldn't handle trying to make conversation with anyone and anyway when my Mum came to visit all I did was hold her hand and cry.

Finally Monday came around and I was informed that as Dr Blake was on holiday Dr Lucas would take the review. I walked in and took a chair. There must have been around eight people in the room and I didn't look at any of them. Dr Lucas asked me a few cursory questions about how I was doing before saying "I gather you've been having some bad thoughts. What are they?"

I took a deep breath, I had only really mentioned the extent of my thoughts to my Mum and this would be the first time that I would speak them out loud to a doctor.

"I'm a terribly evil person and I'm going to burn in Hell."

No response. I looked up and they were all busy writing on their notepads. No one said "No you're not." Which wouldn't really have helped but would at the very least have given me a moment's reassurance. Pause.

"Anything else?"

"The nurses are plotting to harm me. And my parents are planning to throw me out of their house. I'll have to live homeless and destitute for the rest of my life. And…"

"Yes?"

"And there's nothing wrong with me. I'm not ill. You've got it all wrong."

"I see."

"I want to stop taking my antipsychotic. I don't think it's helping me, in fact I think it's making me worse."

"Yes, I agree with you on that point, Suzy. But we'll have to take you off it gradually over a space of three weeks. You can't just stop taking it immediately. That's not the way it works. We'll also gradually introduce another antipsychotic into your medication regime as I think it's important that you're taking one. Okay?"

I felt totally deflated. "Okay." I said in a very small voice.

I had wanted Dr Lucas to stop the antipsychotic there and then but three more weeks? I wasn't sure I could manage that if it was the drug that was causing all of my problems. I could feel its poison pumping through my body and I felt the urge to slice open my arteries and veins and let all the dirty blood flow out of me.

The weeks dragged achingly by and I was getting worse rather than better. The nurses waived the visiting hours for me, and my Mum sat by my bed holding my hand for up to eight hours at a time whilst I cried and cried desperate for some way, any way, to exorcise the demons that were haunting me. I began to lose my faith in the doctors and nurses who surrounded me everyday and seriously question whether I should be taking the medication that they had prescribed for me. Nothing seemed to be helping.

Six weeks into my admission I had had enough and I wrote an open letter to Dr Blake and all of the hospital staff. I read it out in a shaking voice at that week's review. In it I said that I had lost faith in myself, my condition and the doctors and nurses that were trying to help me. I just didn't believe that I was going to get better. This belief wasn't through anybody's incompetence, it was just that I couldn't see anyone, including myself, coming up with any ideas that might help me. I was offered a second opinion but, after talking it over with my Mum, decided to stick with Dr Blake; better the devil you know I suppose and, as ill as I was, I realised that he had my best interests at heart.

Gradually, however, and although I couldn't see it, I was getting better. Everyone was pulling out all the stops to help me – my Mum and Abigail even danced the Sword Dance at the end of my bed one afternoon to make me smile. Unfortunately, when you are in a deep depression improvement isn't always a smooth event. This was the case with me and I began to have wild mood fluctuations from bursting into hysterical laughing fits for hours on end to being in the depths of despair. It was difficult, exhausting and frustrating. In the space of a day I could be feeling depressed in the morning, exultant in the afternoon, and then low again in the evening. I didn't know where I was. My delusions still haunted me, but thankfully to a slightly lesser degree. However, I would be extremely hard on myself to a ridiculous level if I had done anything that I would interpret as "bad". For example, I had borrowed some cigarettes from one of the patients, Eric, and he was discharged before I could repay him. I battered myself with self recriminations and guilt believing that I was a terrible, terrible person for doing such a thing. I would believe that everybody would hate me when they found out and I would be expelled from the Ward. It would usually take a long, gentle talk from Carrie or another nurse, during which I confessed my dreadful deed, before I could bear to live with myself again. This would happen around three or four times a week and I would look for any excuse to condemn myself as an awful person. It was quite a weight to carry around.

One afternoon Mum and I had gone out to enjoy the sunshine and go for a walk to the shops to get some chips. I was feeling good that day and we were enjoying a light conversation as we strolled down the main road back to the hospital. A patient, Jason, had gone missing from the Ward that morning and as we rounded the curve of the bend I saw him sitting on a wall, looking confused and dripping with blood.

"Quick," I whispered to Mum "Go down to the ambulance station and phone the Ward. Tell them we've found Jason and that I'm bringing him up the road."

"Hi Jason! How are you doing?"

He turned to look at me and I saw the razor between his fingers glint in the sun.

"Hi Suzy." He mumbled.

"Do you fancy a chip? I don't think I can finish these." I said approaching him cautiously.

"Yeah, thanks, that would be nice." Standing beside him I could see that there were quite a few deep lacerations on his face and arms and I was nervous of the razor in his hand but I knew that Jason was not the type to hurt other people, just himself, and I wanted to get him back to the hospital as quickly as possible.

"Here you take the chips and finish them if you want. Why don't you hand me the razor and I'll keep it safe for you?"

"No, I don't think so."

185

"Okay then, why not put it behind your ear otherwise you won't have enough hands free to hold the chips and eat them." I wanted that razor out of the way.

"Why don't we go for a walk?" I suggested.

"Where to?"

I took a deep breath and crossed my fingers. "Just up the road. What do you think?"

He thought for a moment. "Yeah, okay." And shuffled off the wall.

We walked up the road back to the hospital exchanging small talk and I noticed out of the corner of my eye that Mum was quietly following us just in case anything bad did happen. As we walked round the bend to the Ward, Carrie was waiting for us. I continued to talk to Jason whilst Carrie edged closer and grabbed the razor from behind his ear.

"Come on Jason, let's go inside and get those cuts seen to." She said taking his arm.

"What about Suzy?" He asked

"I'll come in and have a cigarette with you when you've been cleaned up, okay?" I was starting to shake.

"Thanks Suzy," added Carrie as she led Jason to the door. Then she stopped, turned and said "I'm very proud of you, you know."

Shock settled in later and I had a long talk with Michael, one of the night shift nurses, about the incident when I fully realised the danger that I had put myself in. Perhaps I had acted stupidly and should have waited with Mum at the ambulance station for the nurses to arrive but my instincts told me that if I hadn't done something Jason would have been long gone and up to God knows what with that razor.

CHAPTER 17

The turning point for me was my tenth week in hospital. I got the 'flu and it was the best thing that could have happened to me. I awoke on the morning that I was supposed to go out on pass for the week feeling achy, sick and with a splitting headache. When one of the nurses came to find out why I hadn't shown up for breakfast I said simply "I'm ill." After the doctor had come to see me and diagnosed 'flu it was decided that I could still go home as long as I stayed in bed and rested. So I did exactly that and spent a week sleeping around 18 hours a day. It was exactly the rest that my strained, overwrought mind needed and although physically I felt weak mentally I was much stronger than I had been in a long time.

I returned to the Ward in a much better state of mind and at the review it was decided that I should have another week's pass and if that went well hopefully I should be discharged. I hoped so too. So I went home again and spent a quiet week sitting at home and occasionally meeting up with friends, something I wouldn't have thought possible a few months earlier. Things still weren't perfect, I was still having problems with negative, intrusive thoughts but the new antipsychotic that I was taking had a useful benefit in that as well as taking my required dose I could take extra if I felt I needed to and this helped greatly with any delusions or paranoia that might still be lurking. My self confidence still needed a lot of building as it had taken a considerable knock over the past few months and Dr Lucas, who I had come to trust and lean on, was leaving and was concerned with how much I was depending on her and my Mum. Strange as it may sound my Mum had never met any of my doctors, I preferred to fight my own battles, and Dr Lucas was curious about the relationship between myself and my Mum. I had relied on my Mum's support a great deal during that admission and I think Dr Lucas was concerned that my Mum dominated our relationship. So at my final review Dr Lucas explained that she would see me once a fortnight and in between that she would see Mum and myself for a fortnightly chat to see how things were going.

I was discharged on a wet and windy November morning but had to wait until 5:00pm before I could leave, as my medication didn't arrive from the pharmacy until late afternoon. I was pleased to be going home but a little nervous and apprehensive that the bad thoughts would take over again. I was reassured by a smiling Emma that everything would be okay as long as I took my medication and kept my outpatient appointments. I hugged her goodbye momentarily feeling foolish for ever believing that she would plot against me and think me evil. I got into the car and looked out of the back window until the hospital disappeared into the distance and prayed that my illness would be left behind as easily.

I broke up with Dan for good a few weeks after coming home. I just couldn't shake the left over feelings that he thought that I was bad person and that didn't make for a good, healthy relationship. I was sorry to lose him but I felt it was for the best as I connected him with all of the bad times that I had recently had and I needed to put it all behind me. It was sad in a way as I honestly believe that if I had met him in healthier times we might have been something special but fate decreed it was not to be and so we parted as friends.

I returned home to some nightmarish family problems; my elder brother, Kit, had been going out with my friend from Jordanhill, Liz, for over a year and to begin with I had been delighted and actively encouraged the relationship. But then Liz started behaving in a very strange way. To start with she wouldn't speak to Dan or even acknowledge him when he was in the room. He would ask her a perfectly normal question such as "How was your day, Liz?" and she would reply by picking up a magazine, flicking through it and completely ignoring him. I had had warnings of this type of behaviour a year ago when, after finishing playing a gig in a Glasgow club, she completely lost it with me. The situation had arisen because, after having a couple of drinks with her, I decided that I was going home as I was tired and Ollie, who was there to see the gig, had school the next day and I'd promised Mum we would be home before midnight.

She exploded. So much so, that I thought she was taking the piss and pretending to be angry but then it dawned on me that she really was furious and I dragged her into the ladies toilet as practically everyone in the club was staring at us. It took me forty minutes to calm her down and get any kind of sense out of her. At one point I actually thought that she was going to physically assault me she was that angry. I was stunned. This was a side of her I had never seen before and I didn't like it. Not one bit.

She turned up at the house the next day to apologize which I accepted but a little warning light had been switched on in my brain and I made a mental note to distance myself a little from her.

Things got worse. When I had been in hospital during a previous admission she had come to see me daily and when I had asked her if she would cancel one of her visits because I had a friend from far away who was coming to see me and could only make it at a certain time I received a torrent of abuse down the phone. It upset me so much that the nursing staff put a ban on her coming to visit and also banned any further phone calls from her. I couldn't understand it; she had been a very good and close friend and this sudden change in personality was alarming. I tried to speak to my brother about it but as far as he was concerned he was in love and that was that and he wouldn't hear a word against her.

I had been discharged for over a month and was still meeting with Dr Lucas once a week, fortnightly on my own and fortnightly with my Mum. The meetings were going well and I felt stronger and more self assured as the weeks passed. I think I made it clear to Dr Lucas that whist I leant on my Mum when things were bad I was very much my own person the rest of the time and when Mum was trying to protect me from a difficult topic during one of our sessions I recall Dr Lucas smiling when I said "It's okay Mum, you don't need to wrap me in cotton wool. I can deal with this." Mum and I are extremely close but when I am well I am very independent and more than capable of making my own decisions; it's only when I am ill that I turn to her and others for much needed support and guidance. After meeting with us for a few times I think Dr Lucas began to realise that. I saw Dr Lucas for the last time in the middle of December. I remember that she stood up to say goodbye to me and I thought about giving her a hug but I didn't as I felt shy and awkward. I wish I had and I hope she realises how much I appreciate all that she did for me.

CHAPTER 18

December arrived and my Aunt wanted to have a lunch for my cousin Helen's eighteenth and as my Aunt was recuperating from major surgery she decided that only immediate family would be invited. That was when the shit hit the fan. Liz arrived at my parents' house with Kit meekly in tow and let loose a torrent of abusive language at my Mum and Dad, making all sorts of accusations and calling them a string of offensive names. I was horrified. I couldn't believe that someone could come into a house where they had been made welcome for almost two years and treat my parents like that. It was disgraceful and I was equally angry at Kit for just sitting there and not saying anything. If Liz was expecting my Mum and Dad to explode and make a fight of it she was to be disappointed. When my Dad loses his temper he becomes very calm and icy and speaks in measured, controlled sentences. And my Mum? Well after she had heard Liz's opening tirade she said "It was lovely seeing you again Liz. I'm off to bed. Goodnight." And left the room.

Sitting on a chair in the far corner of the room I was literally shaking with rage, desperately trying to control myself. It all seemed so unreal and I had to pinch myself to let myself know that it was really happening.

"Liz" I said as calmly as I could " I find it slightly incongruous that you can sit there and speak to my parents in such a manner and call them the rude ones."

She turned to me, eyes blazing hate. "Oh yes Suzy!" she spat "You're always so bloody perfect aren't you!"

I can't remember the conversation, if you could call it that, after that. And I don't really want to. All I recall is Liz, dragging Kit along behind her, storming out of the house with my Dad asking Kit to come back tomorrow so that we could somehow sort things out. Liz countered that if Kit was coming so was she. "Oh, great" I thought "Round two."

They came back the next day as promised and had obviously been discussing battle plans as they behaved completely differently. This time both of them refused to talk with Liz avoiding any eye contact with anyone. The only reaction came when Dad, not too subtly to be fair, asked if Liz could go into the next room as he wished to speak to Kit on his own. Liz exploded and shouted that she was leaving, grabbing Kit's car keys and driving off in a fury to Kit's flat at the other end of Helensburgh. Dad, Mum, Ollie and I tried speaking to Kit but it was futile. He kept repeating over and over again that he and Liz were a couple and everything she said was felt by him. I tried again when I drove him back to his flat but he wasn't having any of it. He was in love and that was that. The rest of us had better get in line.

Looking back I feel that that was probably the day that I lost my brother. Up until then we had always been close, looking out for each other and there to help if the other was in trouble. But that was finished and a new, unwelcome chapter had begun. A chapter where I didn't know where he was half the time and I certainly didn't know how he was, he wouldn't let me get that close again. I was to see him one more time after that and that wasn't to be in the best of circumstances.

I spent the following months battling with my inner demons, taking my medication and seeing my doctors regularly. The bad thoughts continued to haunt me and it was only the unerring support of those around me and my pills that kept me from succumbing. Leanne had moved on and was replaced by a new, young CPN called Debra. I was extremely fortunate in that Debra and I got along well and I found her an easy person to get along with and confide in. She was a very likeable and capable nurse and I found her visits helpful. I didn't do much that year, staying healthy was my primary goal and the staff in the Christie Ward had said that it would take me at least a year to recover from the torments that I had endured during my last admission. So I went shopping with my Mum, saw friends and continued to play in the band. I lived quietly and was happy to take my time before embarking on any commitments. However, as the year drew to a close my Mum noticed an advert in the paper for Renfrewshire Association for Mental Health (RAMH) Education Service who were requiring a school worker. I wasn't anywhere even close to being well enough to go for the job but I was curious about what the Education Service did and in the back of my mind I was wondering if they could use a volunteer.

After spending what felt like a large portion of my life being lost in Paisley's one way system I eventually found the Charleston Centre, the headquarters of RAMH. The Charleston Centre is an impressively purpose built modern building which, as I was to discover, has two floors that house many departments from the Education Service, Counselling, REHAB Scotland and many more.

I was met in reception by a bright, enthusiastic and instantly likeable, dark haired woman who introduced herself as Paula Newton. She took me upstairs to the Education Service's office where I explained my background and the reasons for my interest in mental health. I told her how important I think it is to inform young people about taking care of their mental health and also to let them know what mental ill health is all about and thereby reduce stigma. My main motivation for helping though was a personal one. If someone had taken me aside at age seventeen and explained to me what manic depression was and how to get help for it my life would have been easier. True, it wouldn't have taken the symptoms away but it would have given me a better idea about where to go to get help and what could be done about it. She smiled and nodded and explained that the Education Service did exactly that and visited schools in the Renfrew area to talk with 5th and 6th Years about mental health/ill health issues. She also mentioned that they were quite happy to go and give talks to anyone interested whether it be single mother groups, students or school nurses. Paula then asked how I would like to contribute. Nervously I suggested that I would be happy to talk about my experiences of mental ill health showing how good care and appropriate medication can help an individual cope with their illness. I explained that whilst I had really been through the wringer a few times I didn't have any chips on my shoulder and felt that mental health workers, whether they be doctors or nurses, do a great and very worthwhile job. She agreed and added that whilst she was sorry to hear of the rough times I had been through she felt that my experiences could be valuable to others and suggested that I come back in a week and give a ten minute practice talk to herself and Roy, the schools worker. She also suggested that she would sign me up for the volunteer induction that RAMH ran as it would give me an idea

194

of how the organisation worked and might highlight other areas that I might be interested in contributing towards.

My practice talk went reasonably well although I was distracted by other events in my life. I had just heard that Mark, who had become a very close friend during my third admission, had hanged himself. I was devastated. He had been such a lovely, sweet guy who had been unfortunately troubled by heroin addiction, psychosis and depression. We used to spend hours sitting in reception, him with no shoes on, in the Christie Ward talking about what ever sprang to mind. He would confide in me about how worried he was about his thoughts and I would try to reassure him and encourage him to talk to the nurses. He was terribly sensitive to other people's feelings and I remember him taking me aside and warning me that Frank, another patient, wanted to ask me out. He realised that I didn't want to have a relationship with Frank, or anyone else for that matter, but he wanted me to let Frank down gently as he was worried about how he, Frank, would take it.

I also had feelings of guilt about Mark's untimely death as I had promised him that I would phone him when I was discharged. I did call him but he was very short on the phone and I had decided not to call him again for a while. Of course, the next time I did call he had been discharged and I had no way of getting his home number as I didn't know his second name and the Ward, quite rightly, wouldn't give any information out. If only I'd been able to get in touch with him. Maybe it wouldn't have made a difference but at least I could have tried. It also meant that I couldn't go to the funeral and had no proper way of saying goodbye and gaining some closure. I was so sorry. He had been a wonderful person. Bare feet and all.

Giving talks on my experiences of manic depression turned out to be easier than I thought. Of course, I got nervous beforehand but I discovered that I could detach myself quite well from the subject so that it was as though I was talking about someone else. On the whole I seemed to get a pretty good reception and most people felt comfortable enough to ask questions afterwards although I was slightly alarmed by the social worker who asked me how I had caught manic depression! (You can't catch it.)

I also started working in the drop in one night a week which I enjoyed but found slightly stressful as I was putting myself in a situation where I was forcing myself to talk to people. However, the people who attended were generally extremely pleasant and happy to chat away about anything which made things easier for me.

After I had been working at RAMH as a volunteer for almost a year I decided to enrol in the counselling course that the Counselling Service offered to volunteers. I thoroughly enjoyed the course and found it interesting and revealing. I had never thought of myself as bigoted in any way but during the course I discovered that I have feelings of animosity towards people that display stigma against those that have mental health problems. Eye opening stuff! It's something I'm going to have to work on. The course was intensive and demanding; we finished each day like bleary-eyed zombies, so I was both pleased and proud to complete it and be asked if I would be interested in filling a position as a volunteer counsellor. My gut instinct said "Hold on a minute, Suzy" but I was sick of always holding back and desperate to move forward in my life. This seemed like a good way to go so I agreed to take on some clients and see how things progressed.

I was due to see my first client just before Christmas and unfortunately I didn't feel that it went too well. The lady I saw was very upset and cried all the way through the session. I did my best to help her by being positive and empathetic but I didn't feel as though I had reached her and I think both of us left the session feeling unfulfilled. I drove home that day preoccupied with how I could have made the session go better. The next thing I knew a police car was flashing its lights at me telling me to pull over. I had been speeding and they wrote me a ticket and told me to hand my driving licence into the nearest police station. Great. I reported to our local police station that afternoon and had an interesting conversation with the duty officer:

"Good afternoon. I've just been caught speeding and have come to show you my documents."

"You've been caught speeding today?" he asked incredulously.

"Yes. Here's my driving licence." I replied.

"But…*today*?!"

"Uh, yes. Today." I was confused.

He sighed. "But it's nearly Christmas!"

I have to confess I was tempted to agree with him and say "Yes, bastards aren't they?" but I buttoned my lip and handed over my papers.

CHAPTER 19

I think I could date the start of my latest depressive episode to that day that I had been "done" for speeding. I was brooding about my, as I saw it, failure in the counselling session and, joking aside, I was shaken up by my speeding charge. That horrible, familiar feeling began to creep its way back into my life. I started to become nervous in the company of people other than my immediate family and thoughts that I was an evil, desperate person began growing like an unchecked cancer in my brain. I spent the New Year, the Millenium, at Dr Grey's house – I had been friends with her family for years – but excused myself at around 11:30pm to drive home and spend the "bells" with my Mum and Dad. It was an emotional moment. There had been times when I was unsure if I would make it to 2000 and to finally be there was a great feeling of achievement. But even at that moment of celebration inside my head I was running, running, running from the ugly thoughts that were starting to crawl out of the shadows and pester me for attention. I was terrified that things were going to go back to the way they were during my last admission. I wasn't sure if I could survive that again. That had taken all of my resources and had been a close run thing. I couldn't go back to that. No way.

I spoke to Debra about how I was feeling and by the time February rolled around both of us knew that hospital was the only option. I was admitted on February 19th and prayed for a short stay and a quick, painless solution to my depressed and confused state of mind.

The Christie Ward is constantly losing and gaining staff so I was saddened to see that both Emma and Valerie had moved on. I panicked slightly. Who would I talk to? No one would ever understand me as well as Emma, of that I was sure. I pushed thoughts of "How could they do this to me?" firmly away with both arms. They have their own lives and lives change. Mentally I wished them all the best and again thanked them silently for all that they had done. I looked up at the bit of paper that was sellotaped to my locker. Named Nurses: Jonathan Greaves and Danni Watson. Never heard of them. Please let them be nice I prayed, please let them be nice. God was listening. Both Jonathan and Danni turned out to be great people and excellent nurses and both spent a lot of time with me helping me sort out the rational from the irrational in my head. I was still bothered by thoughts that I was an evil person and also that some of the nursing staff were, in some way, against me. As a consequence I spent a lot of my time feeling very anxious and I was taking extra medication almost every day to combat this. It was not a healthy pattern to get into and Danni approached me one day to discuss other options that might suit me better and be equally effective in beating the anxiety. We agreed that playing my guitar (the Ward allowed me to have my acoustic guitar in with me) would help and Danni suggested that I try listening to relaxation tapes. I wasn't too sure as any relaxation tapes that I had listened to in the past I had found irritating and not conducive to relaxation. She countered that there were lots of different types of relaxation tapes and she was sure I could find one that would help. Danni also reminded me that sometimes just talking through whatever it was that was making me feel anxious can be a big help so I was not to feel awkward about approaching her or any of the other staff for a chat.

Danni made a big effort to get to know me during the time that I was admitted to the Ward. I was sitting on my bed one day making pictures in my head out of the leaves on the trees outside when Danni walked into the room.

"Hey there. How are you doing?" she enquired.

"Yeah, I'm okay. And you?"

"Good thanks." She sat down on the chair beside my bed. "I was wondering something."

"What?"

"How about you and I go to the quiet room and you can play me that demo of yours?"

I had recorded pretty loud and, to be frank, abrasive five track demo with the Alkahounds during the summer of the previous year. We had been delighted by the results and whilst I was quick to realise that this was not going to be everyone's cup of tea I was still fiercely proud of it and was chuffed when Danni said that she wanted to hear it.

Fortunately the quiet room was vacant and I placed the CD in the Hi Fi and watched as the mechanism slid it into place. I thought for a second and then selected the most tuneful, non aggressive track for Danni to listen to. I listened for a few seconds before turning to Danni to see what she thought of it. Her expression was a dead giveaway. She quite obviously hated it. I started to chuckle and in an extremely polite voice asked her if she'd like to listen to another track?

"Uh.." she said looking uncomfortable

"It's not really your type of music is it?" I asked grinning.

"Not really. Actually, not at all. Sorry."

"Don't worry, it was worth it just for the look on your face!"

"That obvious?"

"'Fraid so."

I spared her any further torture and ejected the CD and told her that although she didn't enjoy it I appreciated the fact that she had wanted to listen to it at all. We sat and talked for about half an hour when she was called away and I returned to my bed to reacquaint myself with the trees outside.

I was sitting in the smoke room having a fag and talking with Pat, one of the girls in my dorm, when Danni came rushing through from the nurses' office and asked if she could speak to me.

"Sure." I said flicking the ash off my cigarette. "What's up?"

"Come out into the corridor, Suzy." Danni was looking really concerned.

"Why?" I replied standing up. "What's the matter, Danni?"

I was worried. Danni's demeanour indicated that something was far wrong. Oh my God! Mum? Dad? Kit? Ollie? All of these and a thousand more thoughts rushed through my brain. I suddenly wished I was still sitting down. She walked with me out into the empty corridor, her brow furrowed and said:

"It's your guitar. There's been an accident."

I nearly yelled with relief. "My guitar?"

"Yes, someone put it behind the office door to keep it out of the way and another person, who didn't realise that it was there, opened the door and accidentally crushed it."

My guitar was kept in the office as I wasn't allowed to keep it in my room in case, I don't know, I had the urge to hit someone with it or something.

"Oh Danni" I said relief still sinking in that my all family were okay. "It's just a bit of wood and some strings. It doesn't matter. In fact if I remember correctly I bought it off a friend at Uni for about £10. Stop looking so worried!"

"Are you sure? The hospital will pay for a replacement."

"Yeah, God, I thought it was something serious! You looked so concerned."

"Well we weren't sure how you'd react. I'm pleased you're taking it well."

"Honestly, it was a junk shop guitar. I'm not upset I promise you."

It all worked out extremely well in the end; the hospital gave me some money which I then added to some of my own and on my behalf (I wasn't yet well enough to be given a pass) one of my friends in Sound Control, a guitar shop in Glasgow, selected a fine acoustic replacement. I was delighted, only sorry that the nurses had had to go through so much trauma over my busted guitar.

I received a phone call from my brother, Kit, one afternoon after I had been busy glass painting with the art group. He was calling to say that he would be in town at the weekend and would it be okay if he came to visit? I said of course it would be lovely to see him. After I hung up I wished that I had had the bottle to say "Don't bring Liz". I grew increasingly nervous and agitated as the weekend approached, nervous of what Kit would have to say to me and, above all else, nervous that he would bring Liz. I spoke to Carrie about my fears and she reassured me that they wouldn't let Liz on the Ward so I was to try and not worry. Easily said. All I could remember from my previous meeting with Kit were harsh words and by the time the actual visit came round I had worked myself up into such a state one of the nurses gave me a tranquilliser to try to calm me down a bit. I had also felt that Kit had never really understood my illness and asked Carrie for one of the leaflets on manic depression that the Ward kept for this type of situation.

When Kit arrived, alone, the first thing he did was give me a huge hug. I nearly burst into tears I was so relieved and hugged him back as hard as I could. I popped my head round the door of the nurse's office and asked if I could go down to the tea bar and get a coffee with Kit. That was fine so we headed downstairs, sat down with our coffees and talked about everything and nothing. It was very obvious from the outset that Kit didn't want to talk about Liz or what had happened at home last year. That was okay by me as I was in no shape for a heated discussion. I gave him the leaflet and urged him to read it and clumsily tried to explain how important it was to me that he did. He put it in his pocket assuring me he would read it that night and would be back to see me again tomorrow. As he hugged me goodbye I felt strangely deflated; we had resolved nothing and so much had been left unsaid. I was unsure of what to do.

Kit arrived the next day full of bouncing enthusiasm. He always seemed to think that all he had to do was make me laugh and everything would be okay. It doesn't work that way. And I was trying to make him understand that. My illness is a part of me and by not acknowledging it I felt he was not getting to grips with the person I had become. I wasn't fifteen anymore and I had been through the mire a few times. I wanted him to accept me for who I am not who he wanted to imagine me to be damn it! A big pit opened up in my stomach when I tentatively asked him if he had read the leaflet and he fobbed me off by saying he had read a couple of paragraphs but, hey, he been at the pub last night and guess who he'd bumped into? The pit swallowed me whole and I gave up trying to talk to him about

204

anything important. I couldn't find the energy. So whilst on the surface we were having a pleasant conversation about everyday things, inside I was curling up, unhappy and shut out. This was my brother who I loved to pieces and yet I felt further away from him than I had ever been. He was sitting on the chair opposite me and I still couldn't reach him. It was as though an impermeable barrier had been placed between us. I wanted him to somehow slip into my brain for a few seconds so that he could feel how I was feeling. Maybe then he would understand. I don't know. All I knew was that I felt weak and pathetic for not being able to put everything into words. But words are easily beaten away and he had all of his defences up. There was no way through. I sat back in my chair and gave in to the banalities of our conversation. As I hugged him goodbye I had no way of realising that that would be the last time I would see him. And if I had known would it have made a difference? That is a question I ask myself a lot but, to be honest, I don't think that I could have said anything different. He only wanted to hear certain things and they weren't what I wanted to say. The divide between us was just too great.

I recall saying thank you and goodbye to Danni three times during that admission as I kept on thinking that I was going to be discharged. When I did finally leave it was after a six week stay, a six week stay in which I had again had to battle with delusions and hallucinations. Jonathan and Danni had been a great help, Danni even sitting at my bedside until I fell asleep after a particularly unpleasant hallucination of a large spider crawling through the air towards me.

The hallucinations were upsetting and alarming but they only lasted a short while and then everything went back to normal. Far more disturbing and, well, frustrating were the delusions. Half of me would be telling me that it was a good idea to approach the nurses for help if I was feeling bad whilst the other half would be saying "No! It's dangerous! They're plotting to harm you and are speaking ill of you behind your back. Stay away!" I would become exhausted and confused from the inner turmoil and, of course, the whole thing was terribly self defeating as it prevented me from going and getting the help that I needed. I battled for hours every day with my thoughts trying to be rational and hoping that the truth would come out on top. On top of everything else I had lost my "gut instinct" for what was right and what was wrong so I had no internal guide to help me sort out the delusions from the truth. When I was in the grip of a delusion it would be as real to me as the book you're holding in front of you and that was why they were so hard to shift. But whilst they dominated I had a new weapon in that Danni and Jonathan, like Emma and Valerie before them, encouraged me to challenge my thoughts and question why they were there. So when I started thinking bad things about myself, like I was an evil person, I would sit and ask myself why I was thinking that. What was it about me that was evil? What terrible thing had I done? To my relief I could never come up with anything and whilst it didn't make the thought go away it gave me a little corner of rationality to cling on to and help me fight against the negative thoughts. To this day I continue to battle with these thoughts, for example, if I was having a conversation with someone and they mentioned the words "evil person" to me I would have to be careful that I didn't get sucked into a downward spiral of thinking that they were talking about me. It's easily done.

CHAPTER 20

When I returned home I was pleased to quickly settle back into my old routine of volunteering at RAMH and playing in the band. My routine isn't very exciting and maybe that's why I like it. I take pleasure in the small things like going for a coffee on my own and taking a good book to read or sitting in my room strumming my guitar trying to come up with a new song. I enjoy my life and most of all I enjoy being well so it makes sense that I adopt a lifestyle that places few stressful demands on me.

Life was looking rosy with the Alkahounds: we had been informed that Columbia Records had heard our last demo and were showing an interest in us. They wanted us to fly out to Los Angeles and play a few shows, so our new manager, Fred, got busy organising everything. However, the whole plan nearly fell apart before it had started. I had been told by someone at the American Embassy that as I had a diagnosed mental health problem I would need a visa if I wanted to enter the USA, so I filled out the required forms and waited. And waited. Finally, on the day before we were due to fly out and after numerous phone calls, a letter from the Embassy arrived telling me that I had been refused a visa! Shit! I was a panicking wreck so my Mum stepped in and phoned the Embassy and demanded to speak to the head of the visa department. The lady in charge was very helpful and told my Mum that I had been misinformed; apparently I didn't need a visa at all! I should have been furious but I was just so relieved to be going after all that I couldn't wipe the smile off my face.

January 13th dawned as a freezing cold day and I could see my breath wending its way out into the chilly air. I arrived at the airport and met up with the guys. We were a motley crew, all jackets and jeans with assorted big, bulky guitar flight cases the metal edges of which had a nasty habit of hitting your leg leaving tell tale bruises that would last for days. We passed through passport control and security with no hitches and, rather nervously, boarded the plane. Pete and Rob had never flown before so their trepidation was not unexpected but me? I had been hurtled through the air in a metal box plenty of times, it's just that I was of the opinion that if God had intended us to fly he would have equipped us with proper landing gear.

Fortunately, the flight was smooth and mercilessly absent of the turbulence that causes my heart to leap into my mouth and memories of every Hollywood aeroplane disaster flick I have ever seen rush past my eyes. We arrived in snowy Toronto and on our arrival we were told that we would have to pass through American Customs before we could board our flight to LA. Fine, we thought, no problem and stood in line awaiting our turn to be assessed by a grim, unsmiling Custom's official. It was there that the shit hit the fan. We were told by an extremely unfriendly official that if we wanted to play gigs, even free gigs, we needed a work permit and as we didn't have one he wasn't letting us in. We were stunned, the American Embassy had told us we didn't need a work permit as we weren't charging people entry to our shows. We were escorted through to an extremely intimidating set of rooms where a sign on the wall informed us that we were being filmed. I felt like a criminal and I had to keep reminding myself that we had done nothing wrong. After what seemed like an age a Custom's official came and asked us who was in charge of our group. Paul replied that he was and was escorted away into an office for a grilling. When he returned he said that we had 24 hours to produce documentation that showed that we were here on Columbia's invitation and that we were playing our gigs for free. If we didn't do that we would automatically be banned from the USA for a year. Great. All we could do after that was postpone our flight to LA until the following day and try to figure out how we were going to get the necessary papers. I was tired from the flight and hungry and I confess that part of me just wanted to give up and go home. Luckily the boys were made of sterner stuff and after we got something to eat we checked our luggage into a lock up and started making plans. First of all we called Fred, who had flown to LA ahead of us, and explained the situation. He told us that he would call his sister who lived in Toronto and ask her to pick us up from the airport so that we would have somewhere to stay for the night and he would fax the papers to her son's office in the morning.

Thank God for Fred's sister. She collected us from the airport, drove us to her house, organised sleeping arrangements for the four of us and offered to cook us a meal. I could have cried; it was just so great to be somewhere welcoming and hospitable after spending all of those exhausting hours detained in the intimidating confines of US Customs. I think I was asleep before my head hit my pillow. I was absolutely knackered and too tired to even worry about whether the papers would arrive, as we hoped, the following day.

I awoke the next morning momentarily disorientated and unsure of where I was. Slowly everything clicked into place and, frowning, I climbed into the previous days clothes. As the clothes went on so did the memories of what we had been through yesterday and by the time

I took my place at the breakfast table all of my worries and concerns had returned. Anxiously we phoned Fred and he confirmed that all of the necessary documents had been faxed to his nephew's, Gareth's, office and that we should be able to pick them up on the way back to the airport.

We arrived back at the airport thanking Fred's sister profusely and clutching those all- important bits of paper. Customs was waiting for us and once again Paul took charge and was taken away to be interviewed. Nervously we waited for him, unsure of what to expect. The door to the office opened and the Customs Officer came out and motioned for all of us to go in. He explained that he was going to let us continue our trip to LA but that we were not allowed to play any of the gigs we had organised as all of them required an entrance fee and this constituted payment. Because of this we would require a work permit and as we didn't have one the gigs would have to be cancelled. We were devastated. What was the point of going to LA if we couldn't play? What would Columbia think? Our carefully worked out plans were unravelling before our eyes and there was nothing we could do about it. As we left the office and the prying eyes of the camera Paul turned to the Customs Officer and asked him if anyone would really notice or care if we went ahead and played the shows. The Officer replied that Customs Agents would be going to each of the venues and if we were caught playing we would be immediately deported and banned from the US for ten years. Maybe he was bullshitting, or just trying to scare us, whatever, we just couldn't take the chance and mentally I waved goodbye to our gigs.

We decided that we were going to continue our trip and fly on to LA. Fuck it. Hopefully we could organise some free shows once we got there and the trip wouldn't be a dead loss. You never know it might be fun. Once again we boarded a plane and, after carefully making sure that I wasn't sitting next to Pete, I settled back in my seat and shut out the world with the help of my Walkman. Paul shook me on the shoulder a while later and told me to look out of the window. We were flying over Las Vegas and the neon city shouted "Look at me! Look at me!" From the sky there was no hint of fortunes being won and lost or people getting married on a careless whim, there was just the spectacular man made beauty of a million sparkling lights untainted, at least from this distance, by man's greed and vices. On our previous flight to Toronto we had flown over Greenland's icebergs and I had been awed by their serene, transient beauty. They were blue, not white, and the colour had a depth that souls are made of. I looked again at Vegas, closed my eyes, and thought "Give me Nature every time."

We arrived in LA tired and a little dishevelled but we were given a renewed vigour by the thought that, finally, we were here. Fred was there to meet us and took us by taxi to the Youth Hostel that we were to be staying at.

We spent the next couple of days walking for what felt like miles and still failed to make more then a dent in the sprawling metropolis that is Los Angeles. We were hunting down clubs and bars that would let us play for free and finally managed to secure two gigs, both for the next evening. We sat relaxing that night in an English theme pub that had become our local. I recall feeling slightly annoyed about this: what was the point in flying halfway across the world only to sit in a bar that reeked of home? Surely this was our chance to experience the American lifestyle? Pete, however, can be extremely stubborn and this was where he wanted to be so we better like it or lump it. Paul wasn't too impressed either but we both thought that rather than rock Pete's extremely unstable boat we'd give in and, for the sake of band unity, stay put.

The next evening we clambered into a taxi and headed for the rental shop from which we were hiring our amps and a drum kit for Paul. We loaded the gear into a transit van and made our way to the club that we were due to play at. There are plenty of clubs in Glasgow that boast wall to wall beer soaked carpets and filthy toilets so I appreciated the irony that we had come all this way just to play in another one. The club stank but we were in no position to be fussy, besides there was gear to be unloaded. Then we received the first hint that the evening was going to be a disaster – the rental shop had given us the wrong amps. They had packed three guitar amps into the van instead of two guitar amps, one for both me and Pete, and a bass amp, for Rob. As you can't play a bass through a guitar amp (it'll blow) we had to send the van back to the shop to pick up the correct amp and bring it back. All of this was taking up valuable time and by the time they returned with the bass amp we were already due to be on stage ten minutes ago. As a result we had no sound check and played a vastly shortened set. It was a poor performance; we felt rushed and under pressure, and whilst we didn't make mistakes the sound quality was so crap you probably wouldn't have noticed if we had. However, there was no time to dwell on the shortcomings of the gig as it was time to pack up and move onto the next one. The next club, Lush, was marginally better but unfortunately bereft of an audience and we might have well have been playing in a rehearsal room. "Fuck it" I thought "This is my chance to play in Hollywood and I'm going to

212

bloody well enjoy it!" So we played our hearts out to almost ten people and held our heads high.

The ride home in the van squeezed in between amps and guitars was, for me, the best part of the evening. As we drove through the brightly lit still busy streets of Hollywood we listened to the story of jazz that was being played on the radio. It was the perfect soundtrack as I watched people who would quickly fade into my memory going about their lives in a place that I had only seen previously in films and dodgy TV movies. This was my dream. This was their home. This was special. This was terribly ordinary. The thing that struck me most about Los Angeles was not the fame, the money, the glitz or the glamour, it was the amount of homeless people living there. Sure, there are homeless people living in Glasgow but here there are multitudes of them on almost every street corner of every age, sex, creed and colour. What happened to their dreams? I wondered. Wasn't this supposed to be the land of opportunity? How can a city so rich on the one hand turn its other hand away without so much as a backward glance? I was confused and dismayed – confused that this could be allowed to happen and dismayed that with every cent I spent I was confirming the seperateness of our society. I wanted to scrub myself clean of the guilt and shame that was sticking to me. It was horrifying. And I realised that if it were not for the help of my family, friends, medical staff and social workers I could have easily slipped through the ever widening cracks and found myself, lost and desperate, on the streets. How many of these people had a similar story? I was just so sorry.

The following day we had a day off and Paul and I spent the day together shopping for presents and sampling American cuisine. I had never seen a three layered pizza before. Not sure I want to again. We finished a lovely day with a stunning walk along Santa Monica beach as the sun was setting and I took the opportunity to paddle in the Pacific Ocean. The photos don't do it justice.

We arrived back at the Youth Hostel to hear the news that we were cutting our trip short and heading back home the following day. I was disappointed and Paul was furious. He felt, and I agreed with him, that whilst we were here we should make the most of it and go round visiting every record label, state our case and offer to play for them. It would be stupid to leave without trying. Pete, however, was adamant; he wanted to go home and that was all there was to it.

That evening we were sitting talking in the courtyard of the Youth Hostel and I found myself left alone with Pete. He told me that he felt about an eighth of what he had felt for me before as though this was some huge compliment that I had been waiting to hear. I wasn't interested and felt very uncomfortable so I said "I don't know how you want me to respond to that." And picked up my cigarettes and walked back to the room. I was angry. It was as though he thought that my whole self esteem was dependent on how he was feeling about me! Well sod him! I prayed that he wasn't going to start having feelings about me again. I had just got used to him blanking and ignoring me and I didn't want to go through the whole love/hate process again when undoubtedly I wouldn't live up to his warped expectations and wasn't particularly interested in doing so.

We left for the airport at a shockingly early 4:00am and I said a silent goodbye to LA and all of the dreams it had promised but failed to deliver on as we boarded the plane. After six hours of ever cheerful airplane stewardesses and comforting sounds of familiar tunes on my Walkman we landed, once again, in the icy grip of Toronto.

We had a three hour wait until our connecting flight so Paul and I decided to go through to the departure lounge early so that we would have somewhere quiet to sit. Unfortunately, I had felt the unpleasant depths of a depression come on during the flight and I started to panic as the feelings became stronger and stronger. Paul spoke to me and it felt as though he and his words were a thousand miles away down a long tunnel. I was having trouble making out what he was saying and even more trouble making a coherent reply. It was as though everything was falling apart around me and there seemed to be no escape. Paul suggested that I call my Mum for some advice and I clung to the phone as though it were a lifeline. Amongst many soothing words my Mum reminded me of the time change we had gone through from LA to Toronto and asked me if I had remembered to take my pills. I had completely forgotten and, once I had hung up, took them straight away. It was amazing, within half an hour the bad thoughts, depression and feelings of persecution I had been experiencing all faded away and I was able to convince a worried Paul that I was okay and everything was going to be fine. To this day I am unsure whether it was the medication or simply the act of taking it, the placebo effect, that caused me to feel better, but whatever it was it worked and reminded me of how important it is to take my pills on time.

We arrived back in Glasgow on time and into the welcoming arms of family members. I turned to say goodbye to the boys and gave Paul, Rob and Fred a hug farewell. I went to hug Pete but the expression on his face, as though I was a rather small, unpleasant piece of dirt, discouraged me and I made do with an awkward wave goodbye. "Yeah, screw you too, pal." I thought. The trip had not been a success but I was pleased to have found a good friend in Paul and anyway, how many people in Scotland can say they've played in Hollywood?

CHAPTER 21

Within a week of being at home I found myself in the grip of another depressive episode and this one wouldn't shift. It was as though, to put it bluntly, my head was broken. I felt hugely cut off from everyone around me and, as a result, I was finding it extremely difficult to communicate my feelings and thoughts. I was made of stone. I had lost the capacity for feeling any positive emotions and my feet dragged me through a mire of negativity. I was still hallucinating and the suicidal thoughts that continually badgered me were well on the way to wearing me down. Something had to be done to get me out of this rut. I was slowly suffocating and time was running out.

Weekends have always been a difficult time for me as there is no CPN service and the local medical centre is closed. My only option on that Sunday, when I felt as though everything was falling apart around me and I had reached the end of my tether, was to call Lomond Docs, the emergency GP cover for my area. The doctor on the end of the phone line, Dr Adams, asked me to go over to the Vale of Leven so that we could have a chat. My Mum drove me over and I sat in the passenger seat with my eyes closed trying to shut out the sunshine and the noises that the car made as it raced over the bumpy road.

I spoke to Dr Adams for about fifteen minutes. I have no recollection of what was said. He gave me a piece of paper and sent me up to the Christie Ward to be assessed. I told my Mum what was happening and we slowly turned and headed up the stairs to the Ward. I pushed open the heavy wooden door to the Ward and a million familiar smells and sounds hit me. I felt relief, this was where I needed to be at this time. Here was safety and people that would get me better. Dr Bilono met me at reception and took me through to one of the interview rooms. I tried my best to explain how I was feeling but I felt frustrated as the words wouldn't come out correctly. All I wanted to do was curl up somewhere and be on my own, away from prying eyes and questions. Just leave me alone. After the interview Jonathan came through to take me to my allotted bed.

"Hi Suzy" he said gently "Nice to see you again. C'mon, lets get your Mum and take you through."

"Hi Jonathan" I mumbled

I was lucky to have a four bedded dorm all to myself and once Jonathan had left and Mum had unpacked my suitcase I went to the toilet. Now normally going to the toilet isn't that much of a big deal but on that day it was. I had got my period. This was significant as I had noticed that over the previous few years if I was already feeling depressed the lead up to my period exacerbated things and as a result my symptoms were a lot worse. The staff in the hospital knew this, so when Jonathan came back to take an inventory of my things and I told him about getting my period he burst out laughing.

"Well, hopefully your mood will start to pick up now" he smiled. Then seeing the look on my face said "You will get better you know Suzy. You've been here before and got better before. You can do it and we'll be here to help you."

After I had been checked in and Mum had left I walked round to the smoke room and although I saw a few familiar faces I was feeling shy so I sat down in a seat in the far corner of the room to have a cigarette. I was overwhelmed with misery and suicidal thoughts and felt as though I had nowhere to turn. This was the bottom rung of the ladder, a ladder that I had been trying to climb hand over hand and foot over foot for a long time now. But here I was again slipped back down to the bottom. I wasn't sure I had the fight in me to begin climbing again. I sighed. Maybe, with time, that would come again. I realised that although this was the bottom rung it was a safe, secure rung and everyone on it with me, the staff and my friends and family, would do their best to stop me falling off completely. Besides, this rung had a safety net; it was suicide proof and deep down inside I knew that no matter how much I pondered ways of killing myself in reality it wasn't going to happen.

That evening I headed through to the smoke room for yet another cigarette and Carrie sat down beside me for a chat. I was feeling very nervous about speaking to anyone, patients or staff, and by the time she got up to leave I was dripping in sweat and had to go back to my room to have a shower and change my top. I couldn't understand it; Carrie was great and I had known her for a long time but talking to her was excruciating and I had felt terribly anxious during the entire conversation. I was torn between listening to the valuable things she had to say and wanting to get the Hell away and back to the safety of my own room. I do remember that she asked me if I could see any way out of how I was feeling. After some thought I replied that, yes, I could but it was a long way off. She was pleased by this and commented that that was a huge improvement on my last few admissions and that I was making progress.

I had a rotten night that night. It probably didn't help that I was already feeling stressed from having talked to Carrie so when I had an extremely vivid hallucination on top of that I panicked and pressed the emergency button. The nurses on duty came rushing through and I winced as all of the lights stuttered into life. I explained to my captive audience that I had seen a huge bumble bee crawling through the air towards me. Greg, a male nurse, asked me if it had gone. I told him that, yes, it had. He calmed me down and in a comforting way, as though I was five years old, left the lights on so that I wouldn't be left alone in the dark. I shut my eyes tight, pulled the duvet over my head and eventually fell asleep.

I spent most of my time on the Ward by myself, only popping into the smoke room now and again for a quick cigarette. I felt uneasy about being around the staff or other patients and extremely nervous about speaking to anyone. So I spent a lot of time lying on my bed staring at the trees outside the window noting how different they looked at different times of the day or in different weather. It was a peaceful and calming way to spend the day and I valued the time I had. Once again I had brought my acoustic guitar into the Ward with me and I would spend certain times of the day shut in my room strumming away and quietly singing to no one but the cars parked in the car park that my window overlooked.

I was sitting curled up on the chair by the public phone one morning talking to my Mum when the newest patient on the Ward, a solidly built, tall man with a skin head walked by. He stopped, turned to me, made the motion of playing a guitar and said "Was that you I heard yesterday?"

I put my hand over the receiver.

"Yeah, that was me. I think your room is next to mine, sorry if I was disturbing you."

He smiled.

"No, not at all! It sounded great, I was just worried that I was hearing things! I used to be in a band myself so I love hearing live music. Play louder next time!"

He waved goodbye and walked off towards the smoke room. I finished my conversation with Mum and decided that I needed a cigarette so I headed off in the same direction as my short haired friend. I paused as I stood at the entrance to the room and checked out the situation; the people that I tended to sit with were all together in a group at one end of the garishly yellow room and I could see that the big guy was on his own at the other end. My heart went out to him. I knew from past experience how difficult it can be to break into a group at the best of times but when you're ill that difficulty is multiplied tenfold. So I gritted my teeth, braced myself for a conversation and walked over to him.

"Do you mind if I sit here?" I motioned to the seat next to him.

"Not at all. Do you fancy a smoke?" He offered me a cigarette and looked relieved that someone was actually talking to him.

"It's okay, I've got my own. Thanks though. I'm Suzy by the way."

"Hi Suzy, I'm Jack."

We talked for a while about music; he had played in a successful rock band a few years back and I shared some of my experiences with the Alkahounds. He seemed like a really nice guy and was easy to talk to. Eventually we got onto the subject of our admissions:

"So how did you end up here?" I asked.

"Well, let's see. I've lived the party lifestyle for too many years and right now it's caught up with me. I was always big, party Jack and I guess the pressure of living under that title was too much. I remember sitting on a train when suddenly, like the flick of a switch, I believed that everyone on the train was trying to kill me. I got off at the next stop and walked to a bridge I know hiding from people by ducking between parked cars on the way. I made it to the bridge and suddenly everything became clear: I had two choices – I could either jump off the bridge and kill myself or I could go and try to find someone to help me. Those were the only options. I stood there letting the warm breeze whip around my clothes trying to make my mind up. It wasn't an easy decision but finally, thankfully, I walked away from the bridge and made for the hospital. When I got there I was determined not to leave until I had spoken to someone who could help me. Eventually a psychiatrist was called and he admitted me to the Christie Ward. So here I am."

"I'm sorry Jack, it sounds like you've had a pretty rough time of it."

"No, don't you see? I've been given a second chance. I can start being me now, the real me. Forget all the partying, forget being Mr Popular. I know I'm lucky to be here, it could so easily have gone the other way and I intend to make the most of the help on offer while I'm here. This admission is not a failure in my book; it's the starting point of something new and better and I feel hopeful. I realise, though, that at the moment I'm too fragile to be out there in the real world so I'm going to take my time and get better, properly better, and when that happens I'm going to turn my life around into something I can be proud of. I know it won't be easy, a lot of people will be expecting the same old partying guy to reappear, but if it means losing a few friends so be it. This is the way it has got to be or else I might find myself seeking out that bridge again."

"Jack, that's the most positive, brave thing I've heard said in a long time! Good for you! I really hope it all works out for you and if there's anything I can do to help let me know."

"You helped by just coming over and talking to me. I was feeling pretty lonely and isolated and you've helped push those feelings away. Thank you. So will you tell me your story? How did you end up in here?"

I told him a potted history of my life and explained that I suffer from manic depression which had required me to be admitted a few times. Mostly, however, I was still thinking about what he had said. Being admitted not a failure? Wow. That turned everything on its head for me. I could suddenly see things from his point of view and for the first time I began to feel a little pride that I had sought help when I needed it. Yeah, if he believed so strongly that he would get better then maybe there was hope for me. Jack was unusual, most psychiatric patients are so absorbed by their illness that they are unable to see the bigger picture but as I got to know him I realised that he had a patience and optimism that are normally absent amongst Christie Ward patients. He recognised that he was ill but saw that if he gave himself time to recover and took his medication then there was no reason why he couldn't turn his life around. We became good friends and, when we were both feeling a bit better, we would go for walks to the McDonalds along the road and have great discussions over apple pies and steaming cups of stewed coffee.

Ollie had never come to visit me during any of my admissions. It wasn't that he didn't love me or care it was just that, in his head, psychiatric wards brought up memories of "One Flew Over The Cuckoo's Nest" and he wasn't happy about seeing his beloved elder sister in such an environment. When I had started being ill Ollie was only twelve and it was a lot for him, for anyone, to cope with. Ollie is a very caring person and when he saw the agonies that I was going through he would sit down and talk to me about it or, if I needed space, he would stay away. Whatever, he always let me know that he cared and I am eternally grateful that even with the alienating nature of the illness he refused to give up on me and was always there if I needed him, always accepting me for who I was. My illness affected Ollie and this was brought home when, at school, he was asked to write an essay on what frightened him most. He wrote about mental illness and the terrible effects it can have on the individual and their family disclosing his private fears that he too might develop a mental health problem. I'm pleased to say that he remains healthy and free of any psychiatric problems.

I asked Mum if she could bring over some photos of the family for me to keep on my locker and she said she would bring them over that afternoon. She arrived at around 2:00pm and handed over a photo of Ollie whilst saying "Will this do?" she paused "Or would this be better?" And Ollie strolled into the room with a big grin plastered all over his face. I was thrilled to see him, we had always been close and now that the two of us were adults I counted him as one of my best friends and it was great that he had decided to visit. I showed him around the Ward enjoying his surprise that the place was totally different from how he'd expected it to be. Then Mum, Ollie and I went downstairs for a cup of tea and I reassured him that I was feeling better and that hopefully I should be home in a couple of weeks. He asked if there was anything he could do to help and I told him that just being himself and knowing that he was there for me was a tonic in itself.

Like the rest of my family Ollie always made it clear that he loved me. We are quite a demonstrative family and frequently give each other hugs and kisses which I enjoy and find comforting and supportive. Ollie's love, however, is a little different. He loves me, and I love him, unconditionally. He puts no pressure on me to be well and whilst Mum might say "I hope you're better soon" Ollie just lets me know that he loves me regardless of my mood state and that he will always be in my corner. He's a special person who really understands my illness and the demands it puts on me. He's quite happy to just sit in silence with me and hold my hand just to let me know that he's there. When I am depressed Ollie deals with it quite matter of factly by saying "Your lights gone out. Fancy a cup of tea?" He's my rock and I know that regardless of how I'm feeling I can always turn to him and he'll be there to offer a wise word and support. I'm also very lucky in that he is such a thoughtful, kind person: he arrived at the Ward one day with a magazine under his arm, and as he gave it to me he mentioned that in it there was an article on the Pixies, one of my favourite bands, and he had marked the page with a bookmark. The magazine fell open at the right page and I was overjoyed to see that there was indeed a large article on the band. I was absorbed and almost didn't hear Ollie tell me that I might want to take a closer look at the bookmark.

"Huh?" I said feverishly reading the print.

"The bookmark. Check it out"

I stopped reading and picked up the bookmark. It was a ticket to see Guns 'n' Roses later in the year! Fantastic!

Ollie smiled. "Thought that might brighten your day."

That was so typical of Ollie. He instinctively knew what would cheer me up and he did it with as little fuss as possible. We both share a love of rock music and had missed seeing Guns 'n' Roses the last time they were over in the UK so the fact that he had got these tickets, which were like gold dust, was amazing. But more than the ticket it was the thought that I really appreciated, both for hunting down a magazine with a rare Pixies article in it and for giving me something, a concert, to look forward to. He was reminding me that life was worth living without shoving a lecture down my throat and I appreciated it. He's a great guy who was badly burned by the whole "Kit and Liz" debacle. Ollie made several attempts to hold out an olive branch and keep contact with Kit. He was firstly ignored and then secondly stunned by the hurtful accusations and blame that Kit spat at him over the internet. It was completely unfounded and unfair and Kit should know better. Ollie is a smashing person whom I will always love (even taking into account the fact that he puked over my guitar case when he was drunk one night). I'm lucky to have him as a little (6ft 2") brother and I hope he knows that I will always be there for him too.

I was in the smoke room having a cigarette and a brief conversation with Jack when one of the nurses, Lydia, came and told me that I was being moved to a different room. Initially I wasn't bothered, after all a bed is a bed, but when I was informed that the opposite bed was to be occupied by Tanya, a very large girl with violence problems, I became anxious and pleaded to be allowed to stay in my original room. My pleas fell on deaf ears so I decided that my best form of defence was to pull the curtains around my bed and avoid my new roommate as much as possible. I was now torn; I either spent more time in the smoke room which meant talking to the other patients more or staying in my room in the vicinity of Tanya. What to do? I explained to the nurses that I felt hugely intimidated by Tanya and I was scared of what could happen if I inadvertently did something to annoy her. They reassured me that everything would be okay, that they were there and that, anyway, Tanya was due to be transferred in a couple of days as she came from a different area and was going to a hospital nearer her home. So I began spending more time in the smoke room, at least there I felt safe. But hospital is a funny place, you get to know people very quickly. Everyone is at their most vulnerable and very little bullshit goes on. What you see is what you get. It was unavoidable that I should keep bumping into Tanya, after all the Ward is fairly small and it's impossible to avoid people totally. I discovered that my first impressions had been misleading. True, Tanya could be violent but there was more to her than that. She had a kind heart and a good sense of humour and confided in me that she was terrified of being moved to another hospital because, she said, the place where she was going was full of junkies and there was a big drug problem. I tried to reassure her but ultimately there was nothing I could do. That's just the way things were. My Mum came to visit on the afternoon that Tanya was due to leave and brought her some flowers. It wasn't much, just a small bunch of freesias, but Tanya was delighted and almost moved to tears. No one had ever given her flowers before and it suddenly became apparent to me that small signs of affection which I take very much for granted had been absent in her life. I stopped her in the corridor a little later and gave her a hug goodbye. She hugged me back before announcing that she wasn't

227

leaving until after dinner. "Well sod off then!" I joked, something I wouldn't have dared to do even a few days earlier. She looked at me and a huge grin spread across her face "Yeah, you can sod off too!" She finally left at around 6:00pm and we all stood by the windows in the smoke room waving until the ambulance disappeared around the bend. I stayed by the window and stared out into the nothingness and beyond. I wondered what would become of Tanya, whether the glimpses of a kind hearted, warm person that we had seen in growing abundance would win through or whether her circumstances would cause her to revert back to the angry, violent individual that she had been when she first arrived. I suppose that it is here I should start talking about the triumph of the human spirit over adversity but I wasn't so sure. Tanya was who she was because that is how she needed to be in order to survive in her life. The "nice" Tanya didn't stand a chance.

By my fourth week in the Ward I was feeling a lot more stable and my mood was improving. Of course there were still times when I felt like I had been hit by a psychiatric sledge hammer on the back of the head and retreated to my bed feeling frightened and insecure, worried that people were saying unpleasant things about me and that I was a terrible person. Fortunately, however, I was making good progress and those times were becoming few and far between. Getting better can be a difficult time as my mood would vary from one extreme to another, at least when I was depressed all the time I had some kind of continuity, and it can be tiring and disheartening; one minute I would be feeling great and really hopeful that everything would be okay and the next I was plunged deep into the depths of despair and feel as though everything was hopeless. Recovery from a mental illness does not follow a smooth line of improvement and it is often said that the most dangerous time for potentially suicidal patients is when they recover to a degree that they break free from the mind numbing apathy that can overwhelm and find that they actually have the energy to go about trying to kill themselves.

I met regularly with my Named Nurse, Lydia, and I tried to explain the stultifying fog that swamped my brain when I was feeling unwell. We named it "sludge" and she encouraged me to be patient; I was getting better and the sludge episodes would fade as I recovered properly. Patience was something I battled with; I wanted to be better NOW and tantalizing tasters of feeling well in between depressive episodes frustrated me. Of course, I had been in this situation many times before and I knew how the recovery process worked but that didn't stop me from being impatient with myself and wanting everything to be fine immediately.

I had a situation looming that I was concerned about and I talked it over with Lydia and she encouraged me to bring it up at my review that week. I bided my time and waited until there was a pause in the proceedings before nervously asking if I could say something.

"Of course" said Dr Blake turning towards me "what's up?"

"Well, you see, my band's got a gig on Friday and I was wondering if I could get a pass so that I could play it?"

"Hmm. Who would be there with you?"

"Well, my Mum and Dad are going to drive me there and back and they'll be there for the entire gig. Basically we'd arrive, I'd play, finish and jump straight in the car and come back here. I think it would be a good idea as it would reintroduce some normality into my life and it would be a safe environment. I would only consider going if I was feeling okay and had been doing well all week. What do you think?"

"Well" said Dr Blake twisting a pen around with his fingers "I agree with you. I also think that it would be a good way of introducing some normality back into your life. I'm pleased to hear that your parents will be there, I would have some doubts if it was just you on your own, and I see no problem in giving you a pass for that night. In fact I think we'll extend the pass to cover the whole weekend and if all goes well we'll see you back here on Monday and talk about discharge. Okay?"

"Okay. That's great. Thanks."

I skipped out of the room beaming with delight only sad that Jack wouldn't be able to make it to the gig as well. As the day approached my Mum started bringing my electric guitar into the Ward so that I could practise and when one of the other Doctors, Dr Graham, saw it he stopped in his tracks, turned and said "That's not a Gibson Les Paul Standard is it?"

When I replied that, yes, it was indeed a Gibson Les Paul Standard he asked if he could have a quick shot and when I nodded that that would be fine he reverently stroked the wood and played a few chords. He was in heaven. Reluctantly, he handed it back and wished me good luck with the gig commenting ruefully that I had a great guitar. He didn't have to tell me, I already knew and I didn't have to tell him how much I valued this hunk of wood with a few wires attached – I think he could see it in my eyes.

On the day of the gig I was feeling good and decided that I would go for it. Jamie and Jack presented me with a little teddy bear called

Christie and told me that as they couldn't make it I was to sit Christie on top of my amp so that they could be there in spirit if not in body.

Mum, Dad and Ollie arrived that evening to pick me up and once I had collected my medication for the weekend holding tightly onto Christie, I headed out of the door and climbed into the car buzzing with excitement. By the time we arrived at Strawberry Fields, the venue for the night's gig, it was already dark and the lights of Glasgow twinkled invitingly. I helped dad to unload the car and, with Ollie beside me, walked into the club. As my eyes adjusted to the slightly gloomy interior I saw Pete, Rob and Paul standing in a group near the bar. I put my guitar down and nodded hello to them. Paul and Rob came over to talk whilst Pete was occupied with doing an impressive imitation of pretending that I wasn't in the room. I have to say that I was angered by his manner but I knew better than to pursue it. Why did he have to be such an arse about it? I would have been more than happy to let bygones be bygones and put our chequered history behind us but he just couldn't let it go. I sighed. That was his problem not mine. I shook my head and, chatting to Paul, started to unpack my gear.

The gig went well and I was pleased that despite being a little rusty I didn't make too many mistakes. When I had said to Dr Blake that this introduced a degree of normality into my life I wasn't kidding. Playing gigs was part of my life and I was glad to return to it. But it wasn't just playing the gig that I had to cope with, it was the nerves before hand, the stress of remembering all of my parts onstage and the comedown after it was all over. I was extremely pleased to have handled it all well and come through it with no problems. This gives the impression that I don't enjoy playing with the band but that just isn't true, it's just that I recognise areas in which I am vulnerable and in doing so I cope with them better. I would be far more upset if I didn't let myself play because I was afraid of the stress involved. Standing up and doing anything in front of a bunch of strangers will always be nerve wracking but if you believe that your performance is worthwhile and something that you can be proud of and, of course, something that the audience will enjoy then the nerves and stress take second place. When I stood up on that stage I didn't feel like a psychiatric patient anymore; I felt vital and alive and that was the normality I was so desperate to cling to.

I returned to the Ward early on Monday morning eager to be discharged. However, I was disappointed to learn that Dr Blake was away on leave and that meant that his SHO, Dr Kelly, would take the review. The reason I was disappointed was that SHOs don't normally discharge patients and I was worried that I would have to remain in the hospital for another week until Dr Blake returned. I asked if I could speak to Dr Kelly on his own for five minutes and I was pleased when he acquiesced. At around 9:00am one of the nurses came to get me and take me through to see Dr Kelly. I walked into the interview room and took a seat, Dr Kelly was nearly hidden by a formidable pile of encyclopaedia thick files and took a moment to acknowledge me.

"Hi Suzy, How are you?"

"Good thanks."

"How was your pass?"

"Yeah, it went well."

"Yes. The nurses seem to think you got on fine."

"Dr Kelly can I ask you something?"

"Sure, fire away."

I took a deep breath and mentally crossed my fingers.

"I'd really like to be discharged. I feel that my mood has stabilised and I'm not so troubled by hallucinations or bad thoughts. I'm not so withdrawn and I'm more comfortable talking to people. If you discharge me I will make sure that I am receiving the appropriate support and care. I will take my medication, I don't have a problem with non compliance and I will do everything in my power to lead a healthy lifestyle and stay well. I just want to go home and I feel well enough to do so."

"Is that it?" he smiled

"Yup."

"Well, it's encouraging and, I'm sorry to say, unusual to hear someone being so positive. I wish more people had your attitude. Do you live on your own?" he asked flicking through my notes.

"No, I live with my parents and my younger brother. They all understand my illness and are very supportive. If you have any doubts you can ask the nurses."

"No, its okay I believe you. Okay, I'm going to discharge you but I want to be sure that you will see your CPN within the week all right?"

"Whatever. Absolutely." I grinned

"Okay. Well, I hope everything works out for you. If you have any problems contact your GP or CPN immediately, got it?"

"Got it."

"Take care, goodbye."

"Goodbye Dr Kelly, and thanks."

Once again I had to wait until around 5:00pm for my meds to be brought up from the pharmacy but I didn't mind; I was going home and I was going to sleep in my own bed and eat food that wasn't prepared in a hospital. Fantastic! On the quiet I gave Jack my home phone number and address and asked him to keep in touch. He gave me a huge hug and promised that he would. I sat in the smoke room all day delighting in the fact that I could without feeling stressed and awkward. Changed days indeed. I took the opportunity to go and thank some of the nurses that had helped me so much during that admission especially Jonathan, Lydia and Carrie. Sure, they are just doing their job but if it wasn't for their common sense, wisdom and care I don't know how things would have worked out for me. It's easy to take them for granted and I wanted them to know how much I valued their input. I have no doubts that it is because of them, and other doctors and nurses over the past few years, that I am still alive and it doesn't come much blacker or whiter than that.

Mum was waiting for me in the reception when the meds finally turned up and after I had said goodbye to everyone we walked down the stairs and out into the rain. We climbed into the car, buckled up and drove away from my sixth admission down a road that only a few weeks ago had seemed filled with despair and fear but now held the promise of something better; happiness and that most elusive of fellows, hope.

EPILOGUE

I have been out of hospital for over three years now and feel that things are pretty stable. Yes, I still have times of ill health, only this afternoon I was sure that the police were after me (they weren't) and I felt frightened and persecuted but I am getting better at realising when these things are in my head and, as a consequence, take appropriate action. Along with my regular medications I have what is known as a PRN which is a medication (in my case an antipsychotic) that can be taken when required. So this afternoon, once I realised things were getting out of control I had the insight to take a PRN and phone my Mum for some comforting, rational words. In this way I get through the occasional little crisis that can crop up in my life and whilst it isn't perfect it is a big improvement on how I used to handle things just a few years ago. Back then I used to keep everything to myself and I was too scared to let anyone in. I realise now that an objective viewpoint can be helpful although obviously I am careful about who I approach for help as the wrong reaction can do more harm than good. I am extremely lucky in that I can go to my professional network, family and certain friends and tell them anything armed with the knowledge that they won't be shocked or turn me away and will help me deal with the problem that I am having. I just hope I help them as much as they help me.

A lot of things have changed in my life since my last admission; positive changes I think. I have moved out of my parents' home to a wonderful flat about a mile from where they live. My current flatmate, Mel, is a star and we get on famously. She's a superb artist (although she would argue this) so with me writing music and her painting and drawing our flat is quite a little hive of creativity! I'm having a great time living in my flat especially now that I have a rather, to put it politely, eccentric cat to keep me occupied when Mel's out at work. She, Casey, has the rather amusing habit of falling in the bath when I am bathing! The look on her face when this happens is hysterical and she never seems to learn! She is a Tonkinese (Burmese/Siamese cross) and as such is very vocal and affectionate – we have long conversations and I'm only glad that my psychiatrist isn't around to witness them!

One lovely asset of my flat is that it is situated at the front of Helensburgh and looks out over the Clyde. I can sit for hours at the window seat just staring at the water losing myself in the ebb and flow of the tide, careless thoughts drifting through my head like contorted pieces of driftwood washed up on the beach. To be honest the water isn't the cleanest but sometimes I feel the urge to walk into the river and immerse myself in it, drowning out the negative thoughts that continue to plague me and emerge refreshed, cleansed and somehow free of all my problems. I wish.

Well, the inevitable finally happened; Pete kicked me, and surprisingly Paul, out of the Alkahounds. Typically of Pete it was done in a particularly unpleasant and shifty way: he told Paul that the band had split and could he pass on the word to me. He didn't even have the decency to tell me himself. However, Ollie checked the Alkahounds website and reported that on it Pete was boasting about having "dropped the dead weight" and that the band was going from strength to strength. Nice. To be honest it was a relief, I was sick of Pete's shenanigans and even the music wasn't enough to make me want to stay. So Paul and I recruited a singer/guitarist, Lindsay, who

236

is absolutely amazing vocally and on guitar and we've been lucky to find Kenny who is a great bass player. Playing in this band (The Upstares) has been a revelation for me. This is how it is supposed to be when you're in a band: fun! There were no longer any moody silences, bad vibes or blank stares just four musicians getting together and playing for the sheer Hell of it. If you add in the good natured banter between the four of us it becomes clear why, after years of being nervous about rehearsals, I am enjoying myself again. I have no illusions about becoming famous or "making it big", I grew weary of those ideas whilst being in the Alkahounds. No, this band is all about having fun and playing a few gigs here and there. I'm really glad Lindsay is on board as it means that I can just concentrate on my guitar and not have to worry about being the front person and the obvious focal point. I like my anonymity and apart from a few backing vocals I am quite happy to remain in the background.

Recently I came up with an idea that I thought had some potential so I approached Simon and Noreen at The Scottish Association for Mental Health (SAMH) and told them that I felt there was a need for a booklet on mental illness for students. My reasons are such: the most common age of onset for mental illness is between the ages of 17-28 and a high percentage of that age range are in some sort of further education. They agreed and wanted to know if I would be prepared to write the booklet. When I replied that I would be delighted to we discussed things further and decided that packaging-wise it would probably be best to present the booklet as an insert attached to a CD of cool Scottish bands. Noreen has lots of contacts in the Scottish music scene and has managed to get some great bands to contribute and now that I have submitted my final draft of the booklet I can't wait to see how it all looks when it is finished!

On another positive note I am delighted to report that The Scottish Executive's National Programme for Improving Mental Health and Well Being is up and running and I have become involved with the associated "Seeme" campaign that focuses on battling discrimination and stigma. All the people involved, including the Seeme Director, Linda Dunion and National Programme Director, Gregor Henderson, are really positive in their attitude and patiently put up with me calling them with ideas and suggestions! I believe that this programme is innovative and puts Scotland at the forefront of the fight against mental health stigma whilst addressing and promoting all strands of mental health. As one of their volunteers I hope that I have helped to spread the word and I am keen to watch how things progress. Certainly, awareness has a major role to play in making mental illness acceptable and less frightening. With all the writing etc that I have been doing, it was great to be told that I should consider becoming a freelance adviser on mental health. I received further encouragement from the mental health organisations and the Scottish Executive's Mental Health Division and this led to me setting up The Cairn to publish, promote write and advise on mental illness. I am looking forward to this challenge and hope that I will become an asset to the area of mental health.

The only major difficulty that I have been coping with during the past three years has been dreadful social anxiety and I was finding it difficult to go out, and talking to friends was a nightmare. I couldn't understand why this was happening to me - I'd never really had anxiety problems before so what was this all about? After being told

238

that I'd just have to learn to cope with it somehow, I did some research and discovered that the antidepressant that I was taking can, on occasion, cause anxiety as a side effect. I immediately went to my GP, explained what I had found out, and she changed me onto a much newer, reportedly side effect free, medication. The result? Well the improvement has been huge and whilst I still get little twinges of anxiety they are nothing when compared to how things used to be. I am delighted with the change – I am only sorry at all the social events, like weddings and parties, that I missed because I was just too damn anxious to attend. One event that I <u>did</u> go to was my book launch of the original "The Naked Bird Watcher". Sure, I was stressed but I was also nearly moved to tears and flattered by how many people turned up and to hear all of the kind things that they had to say. Thank you all. Mind you, one of the downsides of having written an autobiography is that when you speak to someone who has read it you know nothing about them and they know all about you! Plus, they've heard (read) all of your best anecdotes - bummer!

Another positive thing that has happened is that relations with my elder brother, Kit, and his now wife, Liz, have improved. I made it to the wedding and Kit was almost jumping up and down with excitement and Liz looked absolutely stunning. We had photos taken together and I have started speaking to them both on the phone and they have both been down fairly regularly to see my folks which is a big step forward. I'm looking forward to becoming good friends with both of them again. I have always loved Kit but I feel that we have a lot of catching up to do and I hope it won't be too long before all the bridges are mended.

As you may be aware from first page of this book I have left my original publisher. The reason for this is that as time went on I felt that our personal philosophies on mental health were moving in different directions and I wasn't happy with their set-up either. So I left. I wish them the best for the future but this is one Naked Bird Watcher that would rather be doing things on her own terms and not appearing on websites that were inappropriate and by being there, giving the impression that she was supporting ideas that, in reality, she both disagreed with and felt uncomfortable being associated with. Aside from the anxiety problem (that is now hopefully in the past), mentally I am pleased with the place that I am in right now. I continue to take my medication as prescribed and I see my CPN once a fortnight or more often if required. I have a new CPN, Gary, and we get on well and I find him easy going and easy to talk to. I look forward to his visits as a time to unburden myself of any worries or concerns that might have built up in my head since his last visit. I find this helpful as I realise full well that if I don't talk to someone about these, probably trivial, things they will build up inside me until they dominate my thoughts and cause me all sorts of problems.

Once again February comes round, as it tends to after January, and I find myself depressed and suffering from unpleasant thoughts. The thoughts are a curse and, like nails being scraped down a blackboard, attract your attention for all the wrong reasons. Once again I begin planning ways of killing myself, jumping out of our second floor window held a strange appeal, and become obsessed with the idea that I am a terrible person. Fortunately my doctors are aware of this annual pattern and the strategy is that rather than going into hospital we see how I get on with lots of support and an increase in appropriate medication. Gary, my CPN, increases his number of visits if I require it, whilst my friends are only a phone call away should I need them and should things get worse, I am to return to the doctor's immediately and be admitted to hospital. I don't really want that and neither do my doctors and, so far, I'm pleased to say that after a couple of weeks I have come through it and am delighted that the doctors' strategy has worked. My doctors are incredibly supportive and it is great to know that I can turn to them when I need them. The importance of having family and friends who really understand what is going on, know what to say and do cannot be underestimated, is of huge value and is very much appreciated.

Since then, apart from a few blips here and there, everything has been going well and my life has become delightfully ordinary. Of course, I am careful to stay away from stress as much as possible as I recognise this as a potential trigger for my illness but, unfortunately, in the real world stress is everywhere so I am trying to become better at dealing with it. As someone who used to enjoy and thrive on the challenge of stress, relishing it without so much as a thought, I found the loss of this ability one of the hardest things to get to grips with when my condition developed, and it took some time to recognise there was a real need for me to come to terms with it if my life was to move forward. For the first time in my life I had to start saying 'No' to people and to situations when necessary and will continue to do so if it involves risking to my health. For me, I know the danger of overloading my schedule, so I'm trying to master the art of prioritising. I do my best to stick to a healthy diet – lots of fruit and veg etc and drink plenty of water and, as my medication causes tiredness and being overtired is a risk to my health, I have a nap at some point during the day or early evening if I need it.

So what have I learned from my life so far? I suppose I've learned that sometimes the most obvious clichés are true; there is light at the end of the tunnel and while it may take many helping hands to guide me through the darkness I am lucky that those hands are there to help me when things are at their most desperate. I owe so much to my friends, GPs, CPNs, nurses, psychiatrists and above all, my family. Without these people and their "helping hands" I really don't know where I would have ended up as I'm not sure that I have the strength of character to have made it on my own. It's easy to sit there in your comfy sitting room sofa with your family all around and a good job to go to and talk about people with mental health problems as "them". The point is it is not just "them". Mental illness can strike anyone and statistics show that it does. My Mum has met people who have said to her "But Suzy's intelligent and has a Degree, how can she have mental health problems?" Psychiatric disorders couldn't care less about how smart someone is or for that matter how much money they have or what colour of socks they wear or a million other reasons. All that I did wrong was lose the battle of percentages and develop manic depression. But does that mean that my life is over or somehow worth less than others? I don't think so. And I'm not particularly special, I have met lots of wonderful, caring, intelligent people that cope with crippling mental health problems on a daily basis. These people should be applauded and not talked about in hushed, embarrassed tones. As a society we are ashamed of mental illness and see those suffering from it as weak and as failures. I'm sorry but bollocks to that! Living with a psychiatric disorder can be an excruciating experience not only from the condition itself but also from the potential condemnation by friends and family who can't or won't understand and the strength of will it takes to live with that every day is outstanding. Imagine if you had appendicitis and your friends wouldn't believe you and refused to get you the help you needed and when you finally made it to hospital came to visit only to tell you to "pull yourself together" and "snap out of it". That example may be outrageous and even farcical but how often have I witnessed other patients going through exactly that whilst resident in the Christie Ward? Sometimes you really want to shake people. Snap out of it? Well I say to those people snap out of your prejudice and open your eyes. Statistics show that one in four people will suffer from a mental health problem severe enough to warrant medical care. How many friends do you have?

The best way to fight the battle with mental illness is to arm yourself with knowledge and understanding so that you are prepared and act appropriately if you or someone close to you becomes unwell. It's also important to remember that when a person develops a psychiatric disorder they don't suddenly lose their identity and become "a schizophrenic" or "a depressive", they are still a person with a valuable contribution to make. I don't suddenly stop being Suzy Johnston when I am ill and it's crucial to remember that when you meet someone who is ill to recall that they are an individual and not just a diagnosis.

Depression for me is like walking down a road blindfolded and falling into potholes. You don't know how deep the potholes are or how long it will take you to climb out. The difference for me now is that I know that when I fall into a pothole there will be people on hand to help lift me out. Of course, as you keep walking down the road you may encounter more and more potholes and although I haven't got my climbing out technique perfect yet I'm working on it.

I don't regret the time that I have spent in hospital. I believe that I am a stronger person because of it and whilst I accept that I will in all probability be admitted again at some point I'm not afraid because I feel as though it is the place I need to go to at times in order to get better. And that's fine. However, I am hopeful that the coping strategies that I have learnt over the past few years will help me remain at home and out of hospital for as long as possible. I realise from meeting other patients that my experiences of being an inpatient in a psychiatric ward have been extremely positive and I appreciate how lucky I have been in that sense; I have heard plenty of horror stories. I suppose that this, in a way, has encouraged me to write this book to show that NHS care CAN be effective and helpful. The standard of facilities and care in the Christie Ward are excellent and I only wish it could be more like this across the board.

I have been through some pretty rough times, times I wouldn't wish on my worst enemy but now I realise that even when things were at there worst there was and is always some good that can be taken out of it. I'm not being falsely optimistic just realistic. After all, maybe there's some truth in the saying "That which does not kill you makes you stronger."

I am often asked if I resent my illness, the simple answer to that is "no" because to resent my illness would be to resent the person I have become. These past eleven years of sporadic ill health have given me strength, patience and a will to overcome that I might not otherwise have gained and whilst my life might have been easier and more conventional had I not become ill I have to accept that that was not the way it was meant to be. Life throws difficulties at all of us and it is how we handle them that determines how we turn out. I consider myself lucky, lucky that I have good physical health and people around me whom I love and who love me back. When I am in the Ward I often see people with far worse problems than me and I am full of admiration at how the human spirit can cope with even seemingly insurmountable odds. It can be a humbling experience. More recently I have undergone something of a personal revelation: I can see a future for myself and it is a future that looks bright. If you had asked me just a few years ago how I could see things working out the answer would have been that I would expect myself to be dead before my thirtieth birthday. Not because of a morbid obsession but because, in my mind's eye, I simply didn't see myself being alive that long. Maybe I wouldn't kill myself but my depression might. But now, at least for the present and at age 31, I wake up in the morning looking forward to the day ahead of me and the activities and people in it that make my life so worthwhile. I lean out of my bedroom window and, with the morning breeze on my face, think about those sanity birds soaring gracefully through the air, climbing high in the clear, blue sky and flying out over the endless cobalt sea.

The End

From both patient and carer – rare and unusual insight into mental illness

Two women – One Journey of Recovery
Two Perspectives

The Patient
Suzy Johnston
The Naked Bird Watcher
ISBN 0954809203

The Carer
Jean Johnston
To Walk on Eggshells
ISBN 0954809211

The Cairn
www.thecairn.com

'Suzy Johnston has an incredible ability to both convey her innermost feelings in these experiences and an impartial view of what happened to her - it is that unique ability that sets her and her writing apart'
Doug Huskey, carer, NAMI, USA.

'From Jean Johnston there is now a priceless & refreshingly sensible account on caring for mental illness'
Professor AVP Mackay, OBE, FRCPsych.

'Emotive yet practical, these books should be read by all those affected by mental illness and working within its profession'.
Claire Letham, BSc, RMN, Community Mental Health Nurse.

Available at £10 from all bookshops, internet book sites and The Cairn.

Printed in the United Kingdom
by Lightning Source UK Ltd.
107784UKS00001B/10-12